Conjuring
with
CANNABIS

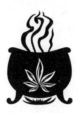

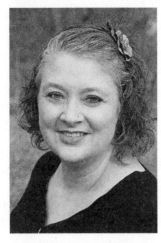

About the Author

Kerri Connor has been practicing her craft for over thirty-five years and has run an eclectic Pagan family group, The Gathering Grove, since 2003.

She is a frequent contributor to Llewellyn annuals and is the author of *Wake, Bake & Meditate: Take Your Spiritual Practice to a Higher Level with Cannabis* and *420 Meditations*. Kerri runs The Spiral Labyrinth, a mini spiritual retreat, at her home in Ringwood, IL.

Conjuring with
CANNABIS

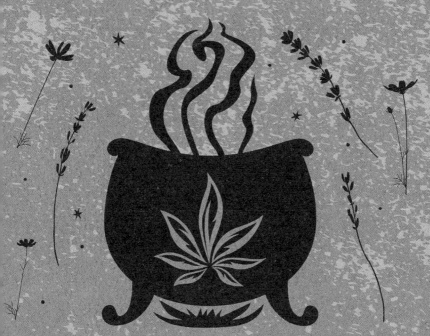

Spells and Rituals for the Weed Witch

Kerri Connor

with Tyler D. Martin and Krystle Hope

Llewellyn Publications | Woodbury, Minnesota

FIRST EDITION
First Printing, 2023

Book design by Samantha Peterson
Cover design by Kevin R. Brown

Llewellyn Publications is a registered trademark of Llewellyn Worldwide Ltd.

Library of Congress Cataloging-in-Publication Data (Pending)
ISBN: 978-0-7383-7270-7

Llewellyn Publications
A Division of Llewellyn Worldwide Ltd.
2143 Wooddale Drive
Woodbury, MN 55125-2989
www.llewellyn.com

Printed in the United States of America

Other Books by Kerri Connor

CBD for Your Health, Mind, and Spirit:
Advice, Recipes, and Meditations to Alleviate
Ailments & Connect to Spirit
(Llewellyn Publications)

Spells for Good Times:
Rituals, Spells & Meditations to Boost
Confidence & Positivity
(Llewellyn Publications)

Ostara (Llewellyn Publications)

Spells for Tough Times (Llewellyn Publications)

The Pocket Guide to Rituals: Magickal References
at Your Fingertips (New Page Books)

The Pocket Idiot's Guide to Potions (Alpha Books)

The Pocket Spell Creator: Magickal References
at Your Fingertips (New Page Books)

Wake, Bake & Meditate: Take Your Spiritual
Practice to a Higher Level with Cannabis
(Llewellyn Publications)

420 Meditations: Enhance Your Spiritual
Practice With Cannabis (Llewellyn Publications)

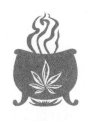

CONTENTS

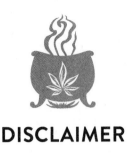

DISCLAIMER

Using, distributing, growing, or selling cannabis is a federal crime and may be illegal in your state or local vicinity. It is your responsibility to understand all laws pertaining to the possession or use of cannabis. Neither the author nor publishers are accountable for consequences derived from the possession or use thereof. Always seek the advice of a qualified health provider regarding medical or mental health questions. This book is not a substitute for medical advice.

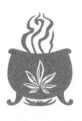

INTRODUCTION

The use of weed in witchcraft is increasing in popularity because it works. Cannabis empowers the practitioner, allows for a greater focus, provides additional avenues of energy, and enables a powerful connection to spirit.

Whether you are an experienced cannabis user or new to the herb, we will guide you along the way to incorporate cannabis into your current conjuring and spiritual practices.

No matter what your tradition or pathway is, cannabis can be incorporated to enhance your spirituality and empower your practice. For rituals and spellwork where an altar is used, set your altar up the way you normally would. The items we tell you to include will be in addition to what you already work with. My main altar always contains representations of the four elements in their corresponding direction, along with representations of the deities I will be working with. Altar clothes, candleholders, bottles, or other containers can all be changed out for different holidays or themes. If I am working an abundance spell, green candleholders may replace my regular clear ones. Specialize everything you do to fit your practice.

With each ritual or spellwork, open and close your working in the way you wish according to your practice. Customize as much as you want. Use your creativity as much as you want. Your altar, spells, and rituals may be simple or elaborate. Build your practice to fit your needs and personality. The more comfortable you are with your magic, the more positive your results will be. If your tradition requires you snuff candles, you may do so where I suggest blowing them out. I am of the mind it releases the energy into the universe to send it to where it needs to go, but as always, if your practice is different, do what works for you.

When we get to our workings, I will use the term *clean* (or a form of clean) to refer to the removal of physical dirt. This includes ash and resin. The term *cleanse* (and its different forms) refers to the metaphysical removal of negativities.

Short and sweet is a stoner's friend; therefore, brevity is used in workings where it is called for. Trying to force your way through a long, dictated ritual while high rather defeats the purpose of the mind-opening journey cannabis provides.

For decades, cannabis was looked down upon as a mind-altering substance instead of the mind-opening plant we now know it to be. Cannabis is designed to work with the body through the endocannabinoid system to produce healing in the body, mind, and spirit.

If you haven't already, please read my book *Wake, Bake & Meditate* to help build your practice. It is the first of my books regarding the spiritual use of cannabis and teaches in depth how to achieve a peak experience. While you will not always need a peak experience for your magic and other workings, there are times when it will be a necessity. *Wake, Bake & Meditate* also guides you along a path of meditations. As a weed witch, meditation and visualizations are some of the most important skills we use in our work.

Tyler is here to lend a hand, especially when it comes to our Herbcraft chapter. Tyler has been researching, developing, and perfecting growing practices for several years. His knowledge has paid off with repeatedly successful harvests. As my assistant at The Gathering Grove, he helps with writing, preparing, and conducting spells and rituals. In his spare time, he enjoys partaking of his favorite muse before writing short scripts he films for YouTube under the name Blue Milk Drinker. We both use cannabis to help get creative juices flowing and to allow for easier channeling while writing.

Krystle joined me in writing *Spells for Good Times* and came back to assist with some rituals and spells. She also writes, preps, and conducts workings with The Grove.

I am an eclectic Pagan witch. As of this writing in 2022, I have been walking a Pagan path for thirty-six years. The more I studied and learned, the more I realized no one pathway was right for me. I felt pulled in different directions, and so my journey took twists and turns with stops along the way. At times, I worried and felt lost because nothing seemed to fit completely. Eventually, I learned that each of the paths I had taken, I had travelled before in previous incarnations. While I didn't remember, my spirit did. Workings I have done with cannabis have reaffirmed this conclusion.

I have spent my writing career focusing on two different topics: weed and witchcraft, and in this book, I get to write about using them together. I love using cannabis with my Craft and have found it to be absolutely, 110 percent beneficial—benefits that you will learn more about as we guide you through this journey together.

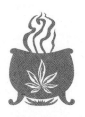

PREPPING YOUR PRACTICE

Before we dive deep into becoming a weed witch, let's go over some of the basics, especially for those who are new to the world of cannabis use.

What Kind of Weed Does a Weed Witch Need?

Cannabis is available in many different forms today depending, of course, on where you live. Some states have cannabis restaurants, but many others are still only at the dispensary stage.

Walking into a dispensary can be overwhelming, and sadly, not all bud tenders are as concerned about the customer as they are about the sale. Having a bit of knowledge of what different products are and about their bioavailability helps you pick out precisely what you need to optimize your experiences.

Products are often broken up into different categories: flower, concentrates, and edibles. Flower is the dried plant buds in their natural state or pre-ground. It can be smoked or used to infuse things such as butter, oils, or alcohol. Smoking is the quickest way to get THC into your system and has the highest bioavailability. The effects from smoking are often felt instantly but can take up to twenty minutes.

Certain concentrates are also heated and inhaled (such as those used through vaping or dabbing). These also have a high bioavailability, and they contain a much higher THC level than flower. Concentrates are not recommended for beginners until they have enough experience in knowing how cannabis affects them.

Other concentrates can be taken sublingually, such as a tincture or Rick Simpson Oil. These will also have high bioavailability. The effects from concentrates are also often felt instantly but can take up to twenty minutes.

Edibles are generally lower doses of THC (per suggested serving), and because edibles take the long route to the bloodstream through the digestive system and liver, the bioavailability is lower. Edibles take longer to kick in, from twenty to ninety minutes to feel the full effects.

It is important to try out THC levels and new products slowly in smaller doses or portions. Experiment and learn how different things affect you. If you are new to cannabis use, or even if you have only consumed by smoking flower, remember, concentrates will pack a much more powerful punch. If you aren't ready for the experience, you may encounter anxiety, paranoia, and even nausea and vomiting. Each type of product brings its own type of energy to your working. Full comprehension of these different types of energies is essential for your weed witch practice. Always understand what energies you are utilizing.

Once you familiarize yourself with different methods, you can learn to layer your THC products in a way that can not only increase but also extend your high to keep you at an optimal level throughout your working.

The type of cannabis you use will affect the energies you work with. Indica carries meditative and relaxing qualities while sativa's energies are focusing and energizing. Throughout most of these workings, you will want to use an indica blend, but when energy raising is involved, a sativa would be more appropriate.

Hitting Your High

Just as different types of cannabis provide different energies, the energy you work with may also be affected by how high you are. The "lower" you are, the more grounded your energies are to the earthly mundane level. The higher you are, the more your energies reach into the ethereal and divine realms, with the desired goal of a peak experience—a peak experience being defined as the period when you feel connected as one, either to deity or the universe around you.

The intention, purpose, and other dynamics of your spell or ritual will dictate what type of energies you want to invoke. For example, if you are a grower and doing a planting ritual, a slight high with a sativa strain will help provide a vigorous, focused type of energy. When you are wanting a deeply spiritual experience, perhaps for shadow work, an intense peak experience from an indica strain would be desirable.

This is where your experimenting pays off. Knowing what it takes to get you to where you want to be for your workings is vital to their success.

Throughout the spells and rituals in this book, we will recommend how high you may want to be for each activity. Remember to keep safety along with your experience level and personal comfort in mind.

Peak Potential

It can be difficult to reach a peak experience; however, there is no doubt in your mind once you have arrived. During a peak experience, you may totally tune out your physical surroundings. You may feel a sudden surge of extreme awareness, with all your senses fine-tuned. You may feel your connection to and place in the universe. Your emotions may become intensified. People often cry tears of love, gratitude, joy, or awe. You may feel as if you spent hours in a peak experience yet come down to find only twenty minutes have passed.

Think about the different ways you use cannabis and how it affects you. Maybe a hit or two calms your nerves, but to get a good high going you may need to smoke several bowls (or repeated doses of whatever form you are consuming). To hit a peak experience, you must go beyond a high while focusing on mindfulness. As your awareness grows, the levels your senses are working at increase too. This includes your sixth sense. If you listen and allow it, this sense may help guide you to hitting your peak experience.

My first indication I am close to hitting a peak experience? I feel my body begin to tingle, almost as if a light electric impulse is running throughout me, making my hairs stand on end. My senses intensify. My normally poor hearing is amplified. If I am outside, the connection to nature becomes overwhelmingly strong. I may at times feel uncomfortable symptoms, such as dry mouth, nausea, or even vomiting.

The first time I hit a peak experience, it was by mistake. I was experimenting and went a bit overboard. I had several friends who told me that smoking weed makes them sick to the point of vomiting. So, I got high and then decided to see what it would take to get me to that point. Not the wisest choice perhaps, but it was this experiment that led me to hitting a peak experience. I got sick and decided to see what would happen next. Again, maybe not the wisest choice at the time, but something inside told me I needed to go further, and so I did. It was then the cool stuff really started to happen.

I felt and saw the opening and cleansing of my chakras, followed by an energy projection of all the chakras at once widening into bright beams of colored lights until they ruptured into embers, like firework trails, each floating off on its own path. A reminder we are each floating around on our own pathways.

As the lights cleared, I felt and saw myself, but not my physical self. My soul self. My higher self. Not as an image but as an energy in which I could feel my connection to everything, no matter what you want to call it: the cosmos, the galaxy, the Force, the All, the One, Nirvana. It was a feeling of absolute peace and weightlessness. Floating. The physical body no longer attached, only anchored. All and yet nothing at the same time.

During my first experiences, I simply relaxed and explored every aspect I could. Eventually, I learned to work with peak experiences for specific purposes, including but not limited to conference calls with my higher self, spirit communication, astral travel, and communing with deities.

The details of your peak may be completely different than mine, or you may be surprised to find how similar they are. There will be both differences and similarities to varying degrees. Do what you are comfortable with and don't push yourself further until you know you are ready.

The bubble of a peak experience is an ideal environment to do shadow work, where your higher self may objectively guide you through the work your spirit needs to accomplish. Peak experiences are not only intended for experienced tokers, but they are also used with workings for seasoned witchcraft practitioners. There are plenty of spells and rituals to gain skills and wisdom from before heading into the more advanced levels of peak experiences and shadow work.

Your peak experience will end when you have accomplished what was necessary. When the work is done, the peak will fade. Again, it may have felt like hours passed only to find it was mere minutes.

If you are concerned about getting "too high," side effects, or want backup in case you find you are not ready, have a friend or partner available to help you out until you are more able to understand your own reactions and processes and can cope with them on your own. You can sniff lemon essential oil, coffee grounds, or coffee beans to help bring yourself down from a high if you become too uncomfortable. CBD will also help counteract the intoxicating effects of THC; therefore, it's a good idea to keep a bottle of concentrated CBD oil on hand—a few drops of a 500 mg oil under the tongue will help curb unwanted effects and bring you back to a more grounded state.

Lit Tips

Two factors to keep in mind while preparing your workings are safety and comfort.

When it comes to safety, if you plan on getting really baked, be sure candles and any other fire sources will be either contained or extinguished. Glass or ceramic cake plates, or other fireproof serving-type dishes or trays, make an excellent addition to your altar. Throw sand (decorative if you want!) onto these plates, add your candles, and you don't have to worry about where the wax drips. This makes burning candles considerably safer, and it allows you more creative uniqueness in your practice.

Depending on the length of the working you are undertaking, you may need to make small provisions for your comfort. Cotton mouth is always a possible side effect. Water and coconut water are refreshing, and mango juice, which is loaded with myrcene, may enhance your high. Whether it's in a water bottle or handcrafted chalice, hydration is important.

If you are a novice at working with cannabis, keep your lemon oil and coffee beans or grounds nearby if you feel you may need them.

Are you prone to munchies when you're baked? Set up a snack tray. Dried and fresh fruits, nuts, cheeses, pickles, veggies, and olives are all easy to prepare ahead of time to munch on throughout your spell or ritual. Since edibles take a long time to kick in, snacking on them during a working may not always be your best option. Remember, eating does have a grounding effect.

Other items you may wish to have on hand include a journal and writing instrument. If you uncover or discover something you want to ensure you remember, you may want to jot it down quickly. Electronic devices can also be used for voice recordings if you are not against bringing technology into your practice.

If your workings include meditations, be sure to get comfy. Use pillows, cushions, blankets—whatever you need to make yourself feel relaxed and at ease. You may want to use a timer or alarm to ensure you do not drift off to sleep.

Spells and rituals do not need to be performed as perfectly as you have seen in TV shows and movies. A little mess, a little chaos, all adds to the authenticity of your work. Always remember, this is your own personal practice, customize it to fit you—hiccups and all.

Elevated Explanations

I use rhymes more in this book than in previous titles because they have a natural rhythm to them that flows well in a baked state of existence. These rhythms will each raise their own energy in easy and sometimes fun and silly ways. Experiment with them. Read them out loud. Try different tempos. Find beats and patterns that work well for you. Give your words additional power by giving them the energy of rhythm and rhyme.

We can be serious and still have fun. Seriousness in our work does not need to be defined by prim and proper behaviors nor solemn attitudes. In fact, it's often easier to raise positive energies while having fun than while in a quiet, somber moment. There is a time for quiet and reflective. There is also a time for loud and rambunctious. How you perform a spell or ritual may change depending upon the type of energy you wish to raise and utilize. As always, do what works for you at the time you are doing it.

Next, we will start pulling together and creating some of the other equipment, tools, and supplies we need to complete the weed witch's cupboard.

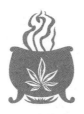

Chapter Two
POWERFUL PARAPHERNALIA

A witch's cupboard contains all their magical tools and supplies, even if the "cupboard" is only figuratively speaking. When you are a weed witch, your inventory of supplies grows. The cupboard of a weed witch may contain rolling papers, grinders, pipes, bongs, and an assortment of other equipment. I have several locations throughout my room where I stash my cupboard items, divided by their purpose.

Next to my main altar, the lid of a large wicker basket creates a base that holds all my non-cannabis smokables, such as mugwort, lavender, and blue lotus flowers. This is where I grind my blends with an old-fashioned hand crank coffee grinder. Underneath my altar is a drawer that contains many of my witchy tools and items, and more are hidden away in the basket.

A lighted case on my wall displays many of my stones and crystals. A celestial-themed small shelving unit holds my oils, a mini cauldron, and other miscellaneous items. A glass double-layer table is home to my to-be-read witchy books, plants, stones, and array of bottles, jars, candles, and other items that take turns on my altar.

The last part of my cupboard in my room contains the rest of my weed witch paraphernalia. This area is set up in two different ways. Refinished, repurposed jewelry boxes keep track of my smaller items: screens, baskets, brushes, spoons, chargers, one-hitters, spare lighters, etc., serving as decorative storage. Next to them, an antique silver mirrored tray serves as my weed altar. This altar contains a special carved wooden box where I keep moon-blessed weed, small jars of some of my blends, a repurposed silver sugar bowl where I keep my ground cannabis supply, an amethyst charging plate, and whichever special pipe or bowl I am using at the time. I have some pieces I use for fun and other pieces I use for spiritual and spell work.

You can build your cupboard in any way that you wish—do what works for you and keep these two important factors in mind: First, you can be as elaborate or as plain as you want with your paraphernalia. You can have one special pipe or you can have ten special pipes. Whatever works for you is what you need. Set up your space how you want with whatever you want.

Second, have fun with it. Be creative. Change it up as often as you want. Add items, get rid of items. Check out your local thrift stores for unique repurposing ideas. Most people don't bother with silver sugar bowls anymore, but for me, they serve as an elegant storage container, holding a place of honor as the focal point of the altar. I have found crystal candy dishes, interesting bottles for making and storing moon water, and other great items I repurposed into my weed witch cupboard. Extra containers come in handy, especially if you grind your own blends. Every witch's cupboard will contain certain staple items. This chapter will help you prepare supplies for yours.

Add a Little Spice

Stocking basic supplies and cleansing equipment for your cupboard will require several rituals and spells. This means you already have several ways in which to experiment with and practice combining cannabis with magic since these are workings that will be performed over and over again as you replenish and cleanse.

How high you want to be is entirely up to you as well as the amount of energy and type of energy you want to contribute to each of these workings. Think about this: if you smoke or otherwise consume an indica strain and are in a dreamy, ethereal-like state, the energy you attach to your moon water will be different than if you use a sativa strain and are drumming and enthusiastically chanting your blessing under the same full moon.

Novices learning how to bless and harness and direct energies may want to keep things on the lighter side. As you become more adept, heightening your high will intensify your experience and outcome. Work at the level you are comfortable with and where you find the greatest connection to your own power.

Before performing the workings in this section, you will want to consume your cannabis. Later, we will include the act of getting high in some of our rituals, but for now, experiment with and practice getting yourself into your desired elevated state.

Moon Water

Moon water is a vital part of any witch's cupboard. Moon water can be used as a final rinse when cleaning and cleansing equipment. Moon water can be used in your bongs and bubblers instead of "plain" water. Moon water can also be used to water your plants if you are a grower.

While most witches use full moon water, you can make and use water from the new moon too. Full moon water holds the qualities of the full moon. New moon water holds the qualities of the new moon. Capture the power of other moons and preserve their energies for later use. Blue moon, supermoon, eclipsed moon—each holds its own power.

Making moon water is a straightforward process. All you need is a translucent glass bottle (with a lid if you desire), clean filtered water, and a full moon or the phase of the moon you want to work with. Pour the filtered water into the bottle and place it outside under the moon.

Focus on instilling your energy into the water. Hold the vessel in your hands and feel your own energy travel down your arms and through the walls of the glass container to swirl and combine with the water. To bless your full moon water, say:

> *Full moon, round and bright,*
> *Bless this water,*
> *I ask tonight.*
> *Fill it with*
> *Your energy and light.*

When the full moon is blue or a supermoon, you can add the appropriate descriptor above: "full blue moon" or "full supermoon."

If you want to make water with the new moon, you use the same process as above but place the water under the new moon.

Again, focus on instilling your energy into the water. Hold the vessel in your hands and feel your own energy travel down your arms and through the walls of the glass container to swirl and combine with the water. To bless your new moon water, say:

> New moon, darkened from sight,
> Bless this water,
> I ask tonight.
> Fill it with
> Your energy and might.

A lunar eclipse holds yet another type of energy. This energy is perfect for wiping the slate clean before undertaking new beginnings and can be especially helpful with certain aspects of shadow spellwork. Capture this energy with lunar eclipse water. Again, use the same process, placing the bottle in a location to soak in the energy from the eclipse.

To bless your lunar eclipse water, instill it with your own energy and look to the moon and say:

> As the shadow crosses your face,
> Your light is hidden
> But not replaced.
> Fill this water with your glow,
> Energy and power
> Of the dark shadow.

If you cannot safely put your water outside, place it in a window. Remember, if the weather is cold, water expands when frozen and can break glass.

Moon Alcohol

If you generally clean your pieces with alcohol and salt, blessing each of these items before you use them provides both a physical cleaning and spiritual cleansing of your cannabis tools.

Moon alcohol is made in the same way as moon water but is used for a very specific purpose—cleaning and cleansing your equipment. This is made with rubbing alcohol instead of water. If you use bong cleaner, you may bless it the same way by placing the cleaner under the full moon. Because we only use this for cleansing and cleaning your tools, you don't need to make it under different phases or moon types, though a supermoon will boost the cleansing energy. Even though you can store moon alcohol (or cleaner) from any moon, when there is a supermoon, you may want to make as many bottles as possible for the extra boost.

To bless your moon alcohol or cleaner, focus on instilling your energy into it. Hold the container in your hands and visualize your own energy traveling down your arms and into the container. Say:

Spirit of the moon above,
Send your energy down

To the spirit in this glass contained,
Your power shall be bound.

Place the bottle either outside or in a window.

Salt Blessing

If you use salt to clean your equipment, bless it ahead of time to use in your cleansing ritual. If you don't normally use salt, adding it gives both your cleansing and cleaning a boost. You may bless your salt in its original container or transfer it to one that is more pleasing to you. I use regular table salt for normal cleaning of my bongs, but when I want to do a ritual cleanse, I pour it into a spouted bottle or pitcher for aesthetic purposes while keeping it easy to pour the salt into bongs or bubblers. This is one of those supplies that can be found by repurposing other items. Most of my containers are thrift store finds.

Because salt is itself a cleansing tool, you only need to bless it with your intention. Your intention in this case is to add a positive energy to the salt to help cleanse away any negative residue on your pieces or tools.

To bless your salt, stand outside with the salt-filled container in your hands, holding it comfortably in front of you. If your container has a lid, leave it open for now so the salt is exposed. Visualize different natural, positive energies in the area around you. Energies in the air, energies from nearby trees and other plants. See the energies radiating all around you. Call to them, harness them, sucking them in through your skin or chakras to travel down your arms, through your fingers, into the container where it blends in swirls throughout the salt.

As you call in this energy, say:

The energies I call upon
To assist me with my will,
I infuse into this salt.

You may chant this repeatedly if you like. Remember to visualize infusing your own energy too. Continue your visualization until you feel it is complete, with the energies blending and settling, becoming one with the grains of salt.

EQUIPMENT CLEANSING AND BLESSING RITUAL

New equipment should be cleansed and blessed before being used and whenever necessary after that. If your equipment is dirty, clean it. If you are preparing for a specific ritual, such as a "high holiday," an equipment cleansing and blessing should be completed as a part of those preparations.

Due to the nature of cleaning and cleansing, you may want to work over a sink, bucket, pile of paper towels, or even outside. Cleaning your pieces can be messy work, so do what works best for you. Personally, I use my bathroom sink and then clean it with rubbing alcohol when I am done to get rid of any sticky residue.

For this ritual you will need:

- Piece being cleaned and cleansed
- Blessed salt
- Your moon alcohol (or moon-blessed cleaner)
- Cleaning supplies such as pipe brushes, cotton swabs and rounds, and whatever else you use to clean your equipment
- Moon water

Open a protective circle if you wish.

Begin by pouring salt into your piece. As you pour, say:

May this blessed salt
Clean and cleanse,
Scour away dirt,
Polish away negativity.

Next, pour in moon alcohol or cleaner. As you pour, say:

Now this liquid,
Blessed by the moon,
Clean and cleanse,
Wash away filth,
Rinse with positivity.

Cover the holes of your piece and shake the mixture inside, adding more salt or liquid if necessary. You may need to do this several times. Each time you add in more salt or liquid, repeat the above. Use your cleaning supplies and clean your piece(s) as needed. As you shake and clean, visualize the positive energies stored in your salt and alcohol scrubbing your piece clean from not only dirt but any negative energies. When finished, rinse once more with the moon-blessed alcohol or cleanser and say:

> *Wash away and clean,*
> *Wash away and cleanse.*

Use your moon water for the last rinse and say:

> *Rinse away and clean,*
> *Rinse away and cleanse.*

If you need to, clean up your area with the alcohol or cleanser and repeat the "wash away" phrasing from above. Follow it with a rinse of moon water and the appropriate phrasing to accompany your work.

End this ritual with "So mote it be" or with your own closing.

MOON BONG WATER BLESSING SPELL

Strengthen your workings by using moon water in your bongs or bubblers. Begin with making your moon water as described above. Save some of your moon water for cleaning and cleansing your equipment, then pour the rest into a separate container to bless for use in your bong.

I use an antique silver teapot I picked up from a thrift store for four dollars. This gives me a beautiful, unique way to store my water with an easy-pour spout. For people who do not like to let their moon water be touched by sunlight, this is also another good option. (As always, you do what works for you and your practice.) Another reason I enjoy my silver teapot is I connect silver with the moon and the goddess; therefore, it is a perfect vessel for some of my sacred water blessed by both.

Whatever container you use, add your moon water, step outside for a better connection to nature (or near a window), and hold it out in front of you.

Just as you did with the salt blessing, visualize different natural positive energies in the area around you. Energies in the air, energies from nearby trees, grass, and plants. See the energy all around you. If you are near water, you can call to those energies too. Call all of them to you, harness them, and absorb them in through your skin or chakras to travel down your arms, through your fingers, into the container where it blends in swirls with your moon water. This practice of calling in those energies and infusing them into whatever you are working with is a skill you will want to master. As always, mix in a dash of your own energy too.

While you work, say:

> The energies I call to aid me in my need,
> Bless this water, which filters my smoke
> To fill my lungs and my body
> With your power
> In each and every toke.

Continue your visualization until you feel it is complete, with the energies blending and settling, becoming one with your moon water. When you are ready to use it, simply pour it into your bong or bubbler as part of your preparation for your working.

CRYSTAL MOON BONG WATER BLESSING SPELL

Crystals contain another form of energy, which can be added into your workings by including them in your moon bong water. Not all crystals can safely be put into water, particularly water that may be ingested or inhaled. Research any stone you want to use first. (By research I mean to look for credible reference information—not just a blog or TikTok, because I guarantee, if you use these for research, you will find contradicting information that can be dangerous and deadly.) Never add selenite, fluorite, or hematite to water. Stones and crystals that cannot have contact with water may be placed next to your moon water vessel, or you may place these stones in a watertight glass container and then drop it into your moon water vessel. Baby food jars are small, airtight, and the perfect size for a few stones to then drop into a pitcher. Glass vials filled with stone or crystal chips also work but be sure the seal is watertight. If it's corked, use sealing wax over the cork to waterproof it.

Once you have chosen your stones, add them to your previously made moon bong water. Again, I use a silver teapot. The teapot has small openings on the inside that lead to the spout tunnel. This prevents stones from getting caught in the tunnel or tumbling out to smack, and possibly crack, a glass piece. Keep these simple hints in mind when choosing a piece to work with for crystal waters.

You will again call energies as you did in the Moon Bong Water Blessing Spell. Calling energies in this manner will become an essential part of your practice. Go outside or stand near a window to visualize the natural positive energies in the area around you. Energies in the air, energies from trees, grass, and plants. See the energies all around you. Call to the energies of nearby water. Call them to you, harness them, and absorb them through your skin or chakras to travel down your arms, through your fingers, into the container where it blends in swirls with your crystal moon water.

As you pull these energies in and infuse your water, say:

> These stones I add to water pure,
> To share their energies, strong and sure.
> As it sits these next few hours,
> Infuse this water with your powers.

Continue your visualization until you feel it is complete, with the energies blending and settling, becoming one with your moon water. Allow the crystal moon water to set at least a few hours (overnight is better) before using in your bong or bubbler.

Crystals for Moon Bong Water

There are several common stones and crystals that are safe to use in your crystal moon bong water, each bringing its own special qualities to the mix. This list will help you get started on creating a cupboard of crystal waters for your practice. Remember, when looking to work with any new stones, do research to ensure they are safe for your purposes.

- **Amethyst** is a versatile crystal. It can help increase your awareness, allowing for greater insight and inner peace. Amethyst is calming and therefore assists in meditation, coping with loss, and settling conflict. It is associated with the crown chakra.

- **Aquamarine** carries the energies of focus, including concentration, discipline, stamina, and honesty. It can assist you in your spiritual growth and pathway to serenity. It is associated with the throat chakra.

- **Carnelian** helps to remove inhibitions, allowing for willingness to come through. This allows a person to feel more helpful, capable, and adventurous. Above all, it is a stone of courage. Carnelian is associated with the sacral chakra.

- **Clear quartz** is an energy amplifier, boosting the other energies around it. Quartz helps to strengthen your perceptions and awareness to bring clarity. It is associated with the crown chakra.

- **Moonstone** helps you to remember your dreams and therefore is beneficial in any dream work. It increases intuition and empathy. Moonstone is associated with the solar plexus chakra.

- **Obsidian** brings healing energies to help with anxiety, pain, and trauma. It opens you up to self-discovery through awareness. Obsidian is associated with the root chakra.

• **Rose quartz** is a crystal of the heart. It opens your heart to love, romance, empathy, and sensuality, and is, of course, associated with the heart chakra.

These crystals and stones (along with many others) can also be combined to create unique blends to suit your needs.

Enchanting Equipment

I have yet to meet a cannabis smoker who doesn't have a favorite pipe or bong they love to use. We all have at least one, if not several. You now have an excuse to buy even more so you may have separate pieces for your spiritual purposes.

Take time to choose your pieces. Listen to what speaks to you. With so many different styles and designs available, it will be easy to find special pieces for your ritual, spell, and meditation work to build your collection.

Crystal pipes are popular, but always ensure the stone you are looking for is not only safe to be smoked from (and not toxic!) but also safe to clean.

Of course, you can also smoke joints or blunts, though I must admit, personally, they aren't for me. I do know many people who like to write their intentions on their rolling papers and wraps.

I have a large bong with the chakra symbols going down the side. This one is perfect for chakra workings and meditations. I have two crystal pipes, including lab-radorite and amethyst, often used in spell or ritual work. My small, silver glass bowl with a crescent moon handle is perfect for my lunar workings.

Your spiritual needs change over your journey, so let your pieces change with you as needed. Always enchant your new equipment with the previous cleaning and cleansing ritual before use.

Your Contemplative Corner

Having the perfect locations for your workings is just as important as your equipment and supplies. While the places you use do not have to be fancy or elaborate, they do need to serve your purposes. You may want to use your bed or a couch for meditations. Or you may take a meditation cushion outside and sit under a tree. In each situation, you need to decide what works best for you. This goes for how and where you set up altars for rituals or spellwork too. You might want to set up inside, outside, in your kitchen, or in your bathroom. I can't emphasize enough how important it is to follow your own heart. This is what your practice is all about—finding what feels and holds true for you. I can tell you how I do things, I can give you hints and suggestions, but eventually, you discover that creating what feels precisely right to you is all part of your journey.

Always keep in mind fire safety when setting up your space to work with candles, particularly when in an altered state. A dish filled with sand, with the candle and holder centered in it, helps keep wax overspills (which cause the flame to grow as the wick becomes more exposed) contained while you are in a meditative state. This is a backup safety measure that can also be decorative, using different colored sand, stones, shells, and other nonflammable items.

Collect your supplies, build your cupboard, and scope out the locations where you want to do your work.

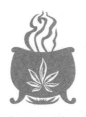

Chapter Three
HERBCRAFT:
SPELLS AND RITUALS FOR
THE GANJA GARDENER

Even if you buy all your products from a dispensary, feel free to stick around for this chapter. You can learn a little about the process of growing, plus see the opportunities for magical workings while progressing through the cultivation cycle, and we will tell you how you can send good vibrations to your own favorite grower!

As with all cannabis products, remember to check your own laws regarding the legality of growing your own. Even "legal" states may have restrictions on who can grow, how much, and where.

Growing your own cannabis is itself a magical process. The transformation of one tiny seed into a plant with dozens of buds filled with healing and connective powers is awe inspiring. When you grow your own, you know precisely everything that has gone into your final bud. You know the circumstances of its growth cycle and life; you know everything there is to know about your plant. This knowledge helps to create a bond between the plant and the grower. As a grower, you infuse your energy into your plants. You also direct other energies into your plants. Once your harvest is complete, your plants return the favor, and you infuse their energies back into you.

The workings we do in this chapter won't require you to be high, but taking a hit or two while working does add to the already-present energies, as discussed in the previous chapter. Put yourself in the state of mind you want to be in before starting your work. When working with sharp instruments such as trimming shears, it may be best not to be too altered.

Whether you grow indoors or outdoors, the first step in growing cannabis is obtaining seeds, so our first step magically will be to bless them.

SEED BLESSING RITUAL

Every grower wants to see big, beautiful, robust buds on their plants at harvest time. To get there, we begin with blessing the seeds for good health and abundance, first with smoke and then with moon water. This ritual includes preparing your seeds for germination to take place.

For this ritual you will need:

- A fireproof container (with trivet if necessary)
- A self-lighting charcoal tablet
- 4 green spell size candles
- A small dish with dried crushed pine needles (about a teaspoon)
- A small dish with a few small pieces of myrrh resin
- A small dish to place your seeds in
- Reclosable plastic bag
- 3 paper towels
- A lighter
- Moon water

Set your altar as normal and place the fireproof container at the center with the charcoal tablet inside. It should be lit during set up to ensure it is ready when needed. Set a candle at each cross-quarter directional point around the container: northeast, northwest, southeast, southwest. Place the dishes in the following order left to right in front of your fireproof container: pine needles, myrrh, and then the seeds. The bag and paper towels should also be on your altar, being sure to keep the bag and towels away from any fire source.

Open your ritual according to your practice.

Light the green candles in a clockwise motion, beginning with the candle at the northeast. Say:

> As I light these candles,
> I call upon their flame to infuse my workings
> with their healing energies and power.

Sprinkle the pine needles onto the lit charcoal tablet and say:

> I pull the essence of healing from these needles.

Visualize the healing essence of the pine needles in the smoke. Pick up the container of seeds and gently swirl it in the smoke above your fireproof container. Say:

> Bless these seeds with your healing strength.
> Infuse your energy with theirs.

Sprinkle the myrrh onto the tablet and say:

> I pull the essence of abundance from this myrrh.

Visualize this essence in the smoke. Again, pass the seeds gently through the smoke. Say:

Bless these seeds with your power for abundance.
Infuse your energy with theirs.

Layer the three paper towels on top of one another and slide them into the plastic bag. Carefully pour the moon water onto the paper towels to dampen them but don't drench them too much. As you work, say:

Water, blessed by the full moon, nourish these seeds.
Grow them through germination.
Give them a strong base to build upon.

Place the seeds on one half of the paper towels and fold the other half on top of them. Squeeze excess air out of the bag and seal it. Hold the bag with the seeds close to your heart; visualize the seeds as they germinate into healthy sprouts. Say:

Imbue these seeds with my energy.
Imbue these seeds with my strength.
Bless these seeds to be fruitful.
Bless these seeds to be healing.

Close your ritual as you normally would. Store the seeds in a cool, dark location while they germinate.

SOIL BLESSING SPELL

A successful cannabis harvest requires the right combination of soils, fertilizers, and other nutrients. Many growers have their own recipe that they swear by for growing their precious seeds into bountiful, bud-filled plants. Whatever your mixture is, use this spell to bless each of the ingredients while you blend them together. Your final blend will be either what you put into planters or work into your outdoor ground soil, depending on how you grow.

For this spell you will need:

- Your choice of cleansing and protecting incense: sage, frankincense, sandalwood, etc.

- Holder for your incense

- A lighter

- A bucket, wheelbarrow, or container large enough for mixing your soil, fertilizer, and other ingredients

- Each one of your mixture's ingredients (If you grow in the ground outdoors, add some of your ground soil to your mixture for this blessing.)

- A trowel (and shovel if working with large quantities)

- If you grow in planters, have those on hand to fill

Begin by setting up your work site. Place your mixing container at a central location. Place your ingredients next to it. You may like to work in a linear fashion: ingredients to your left, mixing container in front of you, empty planters to fill or your garden plot to your right. Set it up in a way that makes sense and works for you.

If you like, cast a circle for your working. I really enjoy incense and love working outside. When I work outside, I like to create a circle of incense around my space with the sticks in the ground.

Light your incense and, using your dominant hand, wave it throughout the container you will be mixing in. As you whirl the smoke around the container, say:

> *Cleanse away anything negative.*
> *All that stays is neutral or positive.*

Wave the incense around each one of your ingredients. (If they are in bags, wave your incense all around the bags.) Again, say:

> *Cleanse away anything negative.*
> *All that stays is neutral or positive.*

Set the incense in a safe place.

For each ingredient, scoop or shovel your desired amount into the container. As you add each one, say:

This mix I make
For bud to bake,
My heart and soul employ.
This mix I make
The mind to wake
To bring me peace and joy.

Once each ingredient has been added, use the trowel, working in a clockwise motion to dig deep and stir your planting medium. As you work, ensuring it is fully blended, envision the energies from the different ingredients mixing and combining, forming into a new whole.

While you stir, chant:

Turn, turn, turn the dirt
With nutrients rich and strong.
Turn, turn, turn the dirt
While I chant this song.

Turn, turn, turn the dirt
For this is what I strive.
Turn, turn, turn the dirt
Help my plants to thrive.

Turn, turn, turn the dirt
Energy I infuse.
Turn, turn, turn the dirt
The plant becomes the muse.

Infuse a portion of your spirit into your blend by visualizing yourself pouring your energy into it while you work.

When you are done, fill your planters or add your combination to your ground soil and work it in. If you were working within a protective circle, close it when you are finished.

COLLECTED RAINWATER BLESSING

Rainwater is a gift from Mother Earth, the gods, the universe—whomever you want to give credit. It is a way to use a less adulterated, less chemically purified water than what comes out of many faucets, and it may help your conservation efforts. It's a more organic, in-touch-with-nature alternative since precipitation is a natural process. Gallon jugs are handy for storing your rainwater and are convenient to work with for a blessing and for watering. If you grow outside or have many plants, you may bless your water right inside of a barrel.

It has traveled a long way, bringing an assortment of energies with it. As clouds form and precipitation occurs, rainwater can pick up pollution we can clean away with a filtering system. Rainwater can also pick up negative vibrations. Negative energy sent out into the universe hangs around until something or someone cleanses it into a neutral state. Rainwater may pass through negative energies and ferry them along the way. Blessing your rainwater with positivity removes any negative vibes it may contain.

For this blessing, you will need:

- Your choice of cleansing and protection incense: sage, frankincense, sandalwood, etc.
- A lighter
- Your collected rainwater

Prepare your location. If you are working outside with a barrel, ensure you can either walk or reach around it. Create a protective circle or other sacred space if you desire.

Light your incense and give yourself a few moments to center. Imagine the pathway your collected rainwater travelled to arrive in your possession. Contemplate the cycle of evaporation and precipitation: water in lakes, rivers, oceans evaporating into the air; the droplets combining to form clouds; clouds releasing precipitation to fall from the sky, hit the ground, and find their way back to a body of water to start the process all over again. This pattern is one of the many cycles of birth, growth, death, and rebirth Mother Nature spins.

Recognize that by collecting rainwater, you interrupt the cycle. The rainwater you collect will nourish your plants, but it won't make it back to a body of water. You have altered its course. You have changed where its energy flows. You have harnessed the energy of the water and will direct where it goes. Be respectful of the energy you have gathered. Honor it for the gift of life it bestows upon your plants. This transfer of energy is essential for plants to survive and thrive. It's also a good analogy for how we work magic: we collect energy and convert it to our use just as we collect rainwater and convert it to plant food.

To continue, swirl your incense in clockwise circles around your container. If it's large, like a barrel, you may walk around it, waving the incense all over. While you work, visualize the energy in the water being cleansed of negativities.

How? Do what works for you. Some people may see the negative energies as a certain color, like glitter, blended into the water. As you cleanse, you visualize the "glitter" being pulled away and disappearing. Others may see the process as big, fluffy scrubbing bubbles dissipating into sparkling clean water. Experiment with different ideas and see what feels right.

While your incense smoke billows around the container, say:

> Water from the sky, which rains,
> Cleanse any negativity it may contain
> So only positivity does remain.

Let your instincts tell you when your work is done. If you cast a protective circle, you may release it. Your rainwater is ready for use to either nourish your plants or be used in the next working. Rainwater can also be used to make your moon water, which we learned about in the previous chapter.

Equipment Cleaning, Cleansing, and Blessing

Growers have a variety of equipment they work with, and this is altered depending on whether they grow outside or inside and in a room or tent. Different growing procedures require different equipment. You may even grow both indoors and out. (I do.) Instead of coming up with all different kinds of ways to cleanse and bless your equipment, we will go over some basics that can be used no matter where or how you grow.

For our purposes here, when we refer to *equipment*, it covers anything and everything you use in your growing process that you would like to cleanse and bless: pots, tools such as trimmers and trowels, lights, fans, and even your grinder. If you have a grow room or tent, it is also a part of your equipment. All the things you need to grow other than your soil, seeds, water, and sunlight can be summed up in your equipment category.

There are three types of equipment when it comes to cleaning:

1. Those you can easily clean with water

2. Electrical appliances (lights and fans), which must be wiped down with a damp towel

3. Those that get incredibly sticky from their close working with the plants and buds (such as trimmers and grinders)

For these last items, you will probably want to use alcohol or bong cleaner. In the previous chapter, you learned how you can make both moon water and moon alcohol and cleaner to use in your blessings. These can be used to clean and cleanse not only your pipes and bongs but also this equipment that needs extra-dissolving power. When you use moon water or alcohol to clean, you can cleanse at the same time with this harnessed power of the moon.

In addition to moon water, you can cleanse and bless equipment with the smoke from different incenses or herbs. You can use incense sticks, dried herbs, or resins on a charcoal tablet in a fireproof container. Do you have a favorite method for using smoke to cleanse and bless? Use it.

My preferred method uses a small cauldron, which can be wafted through a tent or waved through a room and creates enough smoke to pass tools through. Instead of using charcoal to burn the herbs on, I use what I call "Mary Jane magical mulch" and "cannabis kindling" (you will learn about these later in this chapter), and I use a larger cauldron for safety reasons. This helps me to use and incorporate more parts of the plants than just buds into my practice.

No matter what methods you use for cleaning and cleansing, you may choose one of the following chants to recite while working, or combine them together:

For Sticky Work
Clean and cleanse the sticky away,
Clean and cleanse it away.
Clean and cleanse the icky away,
Clean and cleanse it, I say.

Dismiss Negativity
Wash and scrub,
Scrub then rinse.
Negativity I do dismiss.

Refresh and Bless
As I clean,
Refresh and bless,
I set my intentions strong.
As I clean,
Refresh and bless,
I infuse my work with song.
As I clean,
Refresh and bless,
I wash the dirt away.

As I clean,
Refresh and bless,
Only good shall stay.

Soak and Scrub

(Allow the item to soak and then use the
chant as you scrub your tool or piece clean.)
Soak, soak, soak, all day,
Scrub the sticky resin away.

Once you start growing your own, you quickly realize how tacky plants are, and how the resin clings to everything it encounters. Cleanup is time consuming and necessary to keep your tools from obtaining a bunch of buildup.

PLANTING BLESSING

Your seeds have germinated and now it's time to plant them in your blessed soil. Whether you are planting outside into the ground or into planters to go into a tent, we will use the same process.

For this blessing you will need:

- 4 incense sticks of your choice for each seedling. You may want to use cannabis-scented sticks or ones designed for abundance, good health, or protection. Sandalwood, patchouli, or sage are also good options.

- A lighter
- Either your prepared soil in a planter (one for each plant) or your prepared ground space
- Spoon or small trowel
- Your sprouted seedlings
- Moon water in a mister or watering can

Light one incense stick and place it in the east side of your planter. (If you are planting into the ground, work with about a square foot area at a time in a diamond shape. The center of the diamond is where your seedling will be planted. The points of your diamond are the four elemental directions. Place the first incense stick in the east.)

As you place this lit stick into the dirt, say:

> I call upon the winds.
> You who carry the CO_2 plants need to flourish and thrive,
> Bless this seedling with life-giving air.

Light the second incense stick, place it in the south, and say:

> I call upon the sun.
> Your rays carry the power to convert energy.
> Bless this seedling with life-giving light.

Light the third incense stick, place it in the west, and say:

> I call upon the rains.
> You who bring drink to quench their thirst.
> Bless this seedling with life-giving water.

Light the fourth incense stick, place it in the north, and say:

> I call upon the earth.
> You are filled with minerals and nutrients.
> Bless this seedling with your life-giving dirt.

Using a trowel or spoon, dig out a small space for your seedling, being careful not to bump into any of the incense sticks. (Don't burn yourself.)

Gently plant the seedling into the dirt, covering it where needed, and say:

> Into this soil
> Your roots will grow,
> Then into buds
> Your magic will flow.

Visualize sending energy to the seedling as you plant it into the soil.

Use your moon water (a mister is perfect!) to dampen the soil around the seedling and say:

> *I add this water,*
> *Blessed by the moon,*
> *To help ensure*
> *A gardener's boon.*

Leave the incense to burn out around each plant, surrounding it with a protective barrier while you move on to the next plant. Remember to remove the sticks when they are done burning.

CLONES

Clones consist of taking a branch from one plant and giving it a life all its own. When we take a branch to clone, we first give thanks to the mother plant for giving of herself to create a new plant. Her sacrifice gives the gardener a shorter growing time and lets them easily replicate a favorite strain.

Though the clone will have acquired the same blessings as the mother plant since it was once a part of the mother plant, an additional blessing is warranted due to the stress inflicted upon a clone when it is taken from its mother.

Rooting hormones encourage the growth of a root system for a clone, but until one develops, the clone is in a weakened state. Because of the shock of suddenly being cut from its mother plant and left in a fragile condition, clones need extra care, both physically and energetically, to reestablish healthy growth.

For this blessing you will need:

- Your mother plant (not yet budding)
- Snips or pruning shears
- Vessel filled with moon water for clone to soak in
- Rooting hormone
- Prepared, blessed, soil-filled planter or prepped ground
- Trowel or spoon
- Moon water–filled mister to keep ground moist

Cutting a clone from a mother plant will cause her some distress, but no more than regular pruning does. When we take something, we need to give something back, so be sure to give your plant a nice dose of moon water or even crystal moon water to give her a boost after you take your trimmings. It's true that plants like music, making this an ideal time to play some music in the background while you work.

Before you snip your branch(es), say:

This branch I take to start anew,
And clone this mother plant.

I thank you for your daughter,
And this new life, which you grant.

Snip the branch and place it in the vessel of moon water to soak for a moment. While it soaks, say:

May the power of this moon-blessed water,
Help this plant to grow strong.

Dip the branch into the rooting hormone, tapping off any excess. Use the trowel or spoon to dig a hole a few inches deep and plant the clone, packing the ground tightly around it, ensuring it stands sturdily. Say:

Bless this clone to be bountiful,
With ample buds plentiful.

Repeat the process for each clone you cut and plant. Give the soil of each plant a good drenching with your moon water–filled mister to welcome them to their new home.

PRUNING CHANT

Pruning your plants by removing certain branches and leaves keeps them healthy and redirects nutrients to the buds, helping them to grow into big, beautiful flowers. Each gardener has their own code for how much pruning they prefer, ranging from only taking dead leaves to those who trim off as much as possible. Whichever methods you use, voice these words as you work. This chant communicates your intentions to the plant and adds a bit of fun to your labor. Think "Row, Row, Row Your Boat."

Trim, trim, trim, my plant,
Remove what you don't need.
Trim, trim, trim my plant,
How I love my weed.

Keep what you prune. Branches can be dried for the kindling we will discuss later. Green leaves can be dried for tea or juiced to add a boost of cannabinoids to a smoothie.

HARVEST BLESSING

Harvest day calls for mixed feelings. Your babies are all grown to fruition. The time and care you have put into them has (hopefully) paid off with an incredible yield. It's time to cut down your plants and hang them for drying.

This little chant helps celebrate the bounty of your plants. Say it before cutting each of your plants at the base of the stem.

Clip, clip, snip, snip,
Gather a harvest of weed.
Snip, snip, clip, clip,
Bounty from tiny seed.
Clip, clip, snip, snip,
A harvest from the gods.
Snip, snip, clip, clip,
A bounty full of love.

After they are cut, move on to the dehydration invocation to bless your plants for safe drying without molding, and to infuse even more energy.

Be sure to dig out your roots, wash them well, removing all traces of dirt, and dry them for decoctions or other uses.

DEHYDRATION INVOCATION

Whether you wet or dry trim, your plants will need to hang upside down to dry or be placed on a drying rack. While you work, invoke the energies you wish to boost in your weed. Do you want to add more healing energies? More calming energies? Focus on the energies you want to raise in your cannabis as you hang them up or lay them out.

While you work, chant the following:

As my plants now come to dry,
I pull [positive, healing, calming] energy from the sky.
I pull it up from the ground,
In the air, and water found.
I send it to these plants I've grown,
Combine them with my very own.
Infuse these buds with their power
To return to me when I smoke this flower.

Each day, waft the smoke from your favorite incense around, over, and under your drying weed. Repeat the chant each day until they are dried and ready for curing.

TRIMMING CHANT

Your final trimming of your buds before use requires a good eye and a steady hand for a bit of precise snipping. Focus your own energy into your work. Call upon any other energies you wish to infuse into your bud as you trim.

While you work, repeat this little chant:

Trim away, trim away,
Seeds, leaves, and woody twigs.
Trim away, trim away,
All grown from tiny sprigs.
Trim away, trim away,

Fill my buds with joy and love.
Trim away, trim away.
Sent from the gods above.

As you trim away, keep in mind, nothing need be wasted—save all your clippings to be used for kindling or Mary Jane magical mulch.

Practical Magic

Big, beautiful buds may be the overall goal of growing your pot plants, but that doesn't mean the rest of the plant must go to waste. There are magical uses for the other parts of your plant you don't want to miss.

Cannabis Kindling

The first two by-products you will encounter when growing your own are the stems and leaves removed when pruning your live plants. These stems are the first source of your cannabis kindling. Allow the stems to fully dry (in the sun if possible) and snap them into a smaller size if necessary. Store them in a location where they will remain dry and open to the air; an open basket is an ideal container for them.

This kindling, along with Mary Jane magical mulch to get it burning, can be used in small amounts in your fireproof container in place of a charcoal tablet. It can also be used in any other ritual fire to add its energy to your working.

Mary Jane Magical Mulch

Charcoal tablets are popular for two reasons: they are supposed to be easy to light and there aren't many alternatives. Anyone who has used self-lighting charcoal tablets knows they are often anything but "self-lighting," especially if they are older. They lose their umph, and getting them to light and stay lit can be difficult. I created Mary Jane magical mulch as an alternative to charcoal tablets and a way to use all the tiny little bits left over when trimming buds or putting them through the grinder. Since I often must relight charcoal tablets anyway, feeding a small fire isn't much different and has a more natural mood to it than constantly clicking a lighter.

Mary Jane magical mulch is, by nature, highly flammable. You must be extremely careful with it and only use a small amount at a time. Your cauldron needs to be of ample size to allow for safe carrying (if you plan to carry it) while a small fire burns. Do not attempt to move it until after the initial combustion dies down to a manageable level.

Once the fire has died down some, you may add any herbs or other things like paper, offerings, or whatever other small items you need to burn.

To make the mulch you will need:

- Mortar and pestle
- All your tiny trimmings, little stems, and leaves
- A jar with airtight lid
- Alcohol with a minimum of 80 proof, or Florida water. The higher the proof, the more flammable it is.

Using the mortar and pestle, break and grind up your dried trimmings as fine as you can and pour into the jar. Begin slowly pouring in the alcohol, stirring as you go to form a thick paste-like substance. Do not use too much alcohol. You want it damp-wet but not soaking with excess.

When you are ready to use it, scoop a small amount into your cauldron and pile on cannabis kindling *before* you light it. Only use a long lighter to light these! The ignition will give you a nice poof of fire, which will quickly spread to the kindling. You can then feed your fire as necessary. Do not use these indoors.

Mary Jane magical mulch and cannabis kindling can also be used to ignite ceremonial fires or other bonfires.

Tea and Juice

Leaves that are pruned from your plants can either be dried, or if still green, they can also be juiced if you have access to a juicer. This juice can either be drunk or it can be used as an ingredient in a spell or potion. Leaves can be dried and crushed to steep a cannabis tea.

While neither the juice nor tea is what I would describe as "tasty," they can be combined with other ingredients to help cover the taste. Cannabis leaf juice can be added to a smoothie to receive medicinal benefits from the plants. The leaves are filled with different nutrients and small amounts of cannabinoids, which our bodies may benefit from. We can also enjoy these same benefits in the tea. Combining the leaves with a strong herb such as peppermint or thyme before brewing will help give it a more pleasant taste.

Roots

Decoctions made by boiling cannabis root have been in use for centuries to treat sore joints and muscles along with other ailments. The roots, like the rest of the plant, are filled with beneficial compounds. Roots can be dried, crushed, and used in your Mary Jane magical mulch.

You can also find creative ways to incorporate them into your practice. The roots from our harvests have been used as hair for Samhain jack-o'-lanterns and effigies for bonfire burnings.

Wands

What better for a weed witch than a wand made from a cannabis stalk? Once your harvest is completely dried, remove all remaining branches and leaves as close to the stalk as you can. Ensure the stalk is dried all the way through.

Using sandpaper, work the stalk as smooth as you like, or if you prefer, leave it in a more natural state.

Decorate your wand to suit you. Wrap the grip area with twine, leather, ribbon. Attach decorative items—charms, moss, crystals, etc. Customize wands for different needs—healing, protection, dispelling negative energies. As a grower, you have access to plenty of stalks to turn into wands.

Sending Out Good Vibrations

For those who don't grow, you have seen a glimpse into the life cycle of those big, beautiful buds we all love. You can see how growers may develop a spiritual connection with their plants. Growing plants from seeds to maturity, particularly ones that can provide you with so many benefits, is a spiritual experience. Plants that are mass-produced by major agricultural companies don't get the benefit of a one-on-one spiritual connection with their caretaker or end user, such as the one created when you grow your own.

You might not know where your cannabis is grown, but you do know when you look to the night sky, somewhere out there under the same moon, there are plants growing buds for you. (Even if in some places those plants are hidden below the roof of a building, they are still under the moon.)

From new moon to full moon, during the waxing phases when we work on building and manifesting, you may either stand near a window or outside to look up into the vast darkness of the night sky. Project and send out positive vibrations to wherever cannabis plants are grown for the market.

As you send out these positive vibrations and thoughts, say either to yourself or aloud:

> *Wherever you are,*
> *Wherever you grow,*
> *Good vibes from me*
> *To you do flow.*
> *I know someday,*
> *You will be mine,*
> *Our body and spirit*
> *Intertwined.*

Stepping outside or up to a window at night to quickly send some positive vibes and energy to your future plant friends is an easy habit to get into.

Now that we have our flower, let's start using cannabis to conjure with herbal blends.

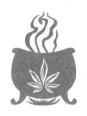

Chapter Four
MAGICAL MIXTURES

One of my favorite parts of working with weed in my magic is including it with smoking blends to help harness and focus the energies I want to connect with. With blends, you use specific energies mentally, physically, and spiritually, allowing for more powerful workings by incorporating the mind-body-spirit triple connection.

While I personally prefer smoking, you might not. There are other ways you can work with blends without smoking them—through the use of teas or tinctures. Each of these methods will also have their own pros and cons.

If you prefer a tea, you can prepare it very similarly to how a blend is prepared for smoking, except you will want to mix together a larger amount of each herb, as teas will use more plant matter. Tea will also have a lower bio-availabilty, meaning it may take a while to feel its effects, and it may take more than one cup of the tea to be effective. You will also most likely need to refresh your cup several times throughout your working. Because of this, I recommend brewing your tea by the potful instead of a cup at a time.

The worst part about using a tea, however, may be the taste. You can sweeten your teas with a natural sweetener, but most may honestly taste awful. Experiment to see what combinations you find the most palatable. Some may be incredibly delicious, but don't expect those results often. Your tea can either include cannabis or accompany another consumption method, such as edibles or vaping.

Tinctures can be made from each herb. This requires a bit of up-front work and time to create tinctures from each of the herbs you want to keep stored in your personal apothecary. Once the work is done, however, it only takes a few drops of each tincture to create your final blended potion. This potion can include a cannabis tincture or accompany another cannabis consumption method. The final product can be taken sublingually for greatest bio-availability. Yes, it will taste bad. Yes, you can use a chaser. Your blend can also be added to a drink. When adding to a drink, don't "water it down" too much. Put it into a small enough beverage to drink quickly in just a couple of swallows; don't draw it out with little sips.

Let's break this down to see how blends work to benefit your practice.

The mental aspects of your workings include your knowledge and your intention. Knowledge tells you the type of energies each herb contains. For example, lavender is calming and relaxing and contains energies that help to calm you when called upon and used. Knowing what lavender does helps you to call upon those energies. Your intention is also a part of the mental aspect as you consciously set and state your wishes or desires.

With blends, you take in the energies, making them a part of you physically. Because of this, it is extremely important to be aware of any allergies before experimenting with blends. Do not smoke or ingest anything you may be allergic to.

The spiritual aspect of your workings is your connection to your higher power or the universe. This is where your beliefs, traditions, and pathway come into play. This is where you connect with energies in the spiritual realm.

These blends offer a complete listing of plants you can include, though you do not need to include them all. I do suggest adding a minimum of three ingredients to your cannabis. For instance, lavender is a fragrant bud, which can also help cover the taste of bitter herbs. Adjust them for your own personal tastes and budget, as some of them can be on the expensive side. Since everyone is different, it is important to experiment and find what blends work best for you, and experimenting can be fun. Learn what you like and what you don't like.

Choose the herbs you want to work with and grind them together. I tend to use equal parts of each herb, grind them together and then add the blend to my cannabis in a 1:1 ratio. I always keep a jar of each blend on hand so that they are available whenever I need them.

This also works for preparing teas. Choose your herbs and blend them together in whatever amounts work best for your needs, ensuring you have enough of the mixture for refills if necessary.

The biggest problem with smoking blends is finding something big enough to smoke them in. While this problem is eliminated with rolling your own, it is more difficult to smoke blends in bowls and pipes and get enough in one filling—combining cannabis with other herbs means less cannabis in each bowl. To remedy this, I either smoke several bowls at once, or I have also rigged a hookah. I do not use the self-lighting charcoal tablets on a hookah. I do, however, have a screen that covers the hookah holes, allowing me to pile up a bit of herb, which can then easily be lit with a torch lighter or hemp wick. Refilling during a session can break your concentration, so figure out what works best for you.

MEDITATION MOTIVATION

Until I began smoking weed, I was terrible at meditation. I couldn't focus. My mind was way too scattered and way too overstimulated. Calming it down to only a few stray thoughts at a time didn't seem possible. Then I learned how to use cannabis to benefit me in my meditation practice. Adding herbs has increased the depth and imagery of my meditations. They help to get me into a meditative state quicker and allow me to stay longer.

These herbs can be used for any of your meditations where another blend wouldn't be more suitable (such as if you wanted to do a healing meditation, then you would use a healing blend). They make a perfect accompaniment to many of the practices in my book *420 Meditations*.

For this blend you will want an indica. Choose from these herbs and grind together in the ratios you wish.

- Blue lotus
- Mugwort
- Mullein
- Skullcap

- White sage
- Wormwood

If you are making a tea, experiment with combinations and ratios for your perfect fit and taste preferences. Tinctures can also be combined in different combinations and ratios.

When you are ready, consume your blend and get yourself into a comfortable position for meditating. If you like to lie down, consider setting a timer if falling asleep would be a problem.

Close your eyes and take several deep breaths. Inhale for a count of four; exhale for a count of four. Allow the herbs to work their magic and begin your meditation.

HEALING HERBALS

Healing can occur in any of several different facets—physical, mental, emotional, or spiritual. Healing in one of these areas can also lead to healing in other areas. These herbs hold healing energies, which can be used in healing across the spectrum.

For this blend, you may want to use either an indica or sativa depending on the type of healing you are looking for. If your healing requires raising energy, use a sativa.

Choose from these herbs and grind together in the ratios you wish.

- Calendula
- Coltsfoot
- Eucalyptus
- Holy basil
- Lobelia
- Mint
- Motherwort
- Mullein
- Peppermint
- Rosemary
- Thyme
- White sage
- Wild lettuce
- Wormwood

If you are making a tea, experiment with combinations and ratios for your perfect fit and taste preferences. Tinctures can also be combined in different combinations and ratios.

When you are ready, consume your blend and get yourself into a comfortable position for meditating. If you like to lie down, consider setting a timer if falling asleep would be a problem.

Close your eyes and take several deep breaths. Inhale for a count of four; exhale for a count of four. Allow the herbs to work their magic and begin your meditation.

Remember how you called upon the energies of plants around you in previous chapters? Well now you have inhaled or ingested the energies of several different plants! Visualize those energies as they move throughout your body. You may want to see them as different colored waves of light—swirling, ebbing, and flowing as they travel along. Send them to where they need to go. Is the healing you need physical? Send the energies to heal the ailment. Is the healing you need emotional? Send the energies to your heart to symbolize emotional healing. Symbolize mental healing by sending the energy to your brain. Finally, for spiritual healing visualize sending the energy to your higher self.

Allow yourself to relax fully and focus on what you need to heal. Ask yourself, what do you need? Allow your intuition and higher self to answer. Do not confuse wants with needs. Your higher self knows the difference, so listen for the correct answer.

Silently say to yourself:

I am healed,
I am whole.

I am healed,
Body, mind, soul.

Experiment with repeating the lines in synchronization with your breathing. Find the pattern that works best for you. Continue your chant and visualization for as long as you feel the need.

ANXIETY RELIEF SPELL

Indica strains are known for helping to relieve anxiety—though some people do have the opposite reaction and they cause anxiety instead. Combining cannabis with these other herbs not only increases the anxiety relief properties, but they also increase the level of relaxation experienced.

Choose an indica strain to combine with any of these herbs and grind together in the ratios you wish.

- Blue vervain
- California poppy
- Chamomile
- Holy basil
- Hops
- Lavender

- Motherwort
- Passionflower
- Rose petals
- Wild lettuce

If you are making a tea, experiment with combinations and ratios for your perfect fit and taste preferences. Tinctures can also be combined in different combinations and ratios.

If you need to settle or recover from an anxiety attack, or if you feel one coming on, consume your blend and get yourself into a comfortable position for meditating. Once you feel a panic attack coming on, the sooner you can work to counteract it, the better. If you like to lie down, consider setting a timer if falling asleep would be a problem.

Close your eyes and take several deep breaths. Inhale for a count of four; exhale for a count of four. Allow the herbs to work their magic and begin your meditation.

Focus on holding your tongue at the bottom of your mouth. Feel waves of calm wash over you, flushing your anxiety away.

You may either think to yourself or quietly repeat the following:

I am okay.
I am safe.

I am calm.
I am at peace.

Experiment with repeating the lines in synchronization with your breathing. Find the pattern that works best for you. You may find you need to start off at a faster pace, which can then be slowed as you transition yourself from a state of anxiety to one of calm.

When working a spell to dispel anxiety, keep your focus inward and control the most important thing you can: your breathing. Focus on your breathing and consciously slow it by counting through each breath. Trying to hurry your way over an attack can increase your anxiety, which could end up extending and possibly deepening the damage. Allow yourself all the time you need to recover. Breathe, slow your breath, and continue to repeat the words above until you feel restored.

Once you have done this several times, it will feel like second nature and be easier to do even if you aren't sitting or lying down. You can learn to head off anxiety attacks as they begin or help reduce your overall anxiety level.

AFFECTIONATE APHRODISIAC

While there is no doubt weed is an aphrodisiac, its amorous and dreamlike qualities can be amplified with the addition of other herbs. Share this blend with your partner for an increased sensual experience.

With this blend you may use either an indica or sativa depending on your needs. Choose from these herbs and grind together in the ratios you wish.

- Blue lotus flower
- California poppy
- Damiana leaf
- Hibiscus
- Jasmine
- Lavender
- Rose petals
- White horehound

If you are making a tea, experiment with combinations and ratios for your perfect fit and taste preferences. Tinctures can also be combined in different combinations and ratios.

When you are ready to use your blend, inhale or ingest while envisioning the energies of sensuality and passion swirling in the smoke in your lungs or coursing through the blood in your veins. See these energies as their corresponding colors—purple and red respectively.

Instead of meditating on these energies, harness them, focus them, and release them in your lovemaking.

SLEEP-INDUCING SPELL

Turn your nighttime hits into a divine, sleep-inducing experience. As a medical user with a high tolerance level, I found smoking cannabis before bed stopped helping me sleep the way it had when my tolerance level was lower. However, tolerance breaks are about impossible due to the massive onset of pain and an inability to function. I learned to increase the effects of cannabis by adding other herbs to it that could also help me sleep.

This sleep-inducing blend was my first foray into working with cannabis herbal blends. My favorite version of this blend includes all these herbs except the catnip (makes me sneeze!). I use it on my hookah and will smoke about two tablespoons before bed.

Choose from these herbs and grind together in the ratios you wish along with an indica strain.

- Blue lotus
- Catnip
- Chamomile
- Hops
- Jasmine
- Lavender
- Lemon balm

- Passionflower
- Sacred lotus

If you are making a tea, experiment with combinations and ratios for your perfect fit and taste preferences. Tinctures can also be combined in different combinations and ratios.

Consume your blend and climb into bed. Lie on your back with your arms comfortably at your sides. Close your eyes and pay attention to your breathing. Focus on holding your tongue at the bottom of your mouth.

As you breathe, think the words:

Sleep for now,
Sleep I vow.

Begin to slow your breathing until you hit a deep, relaxing pace. Slow the words in time with the slowing of each breath. Remain in the now, focusing only on those words as you breathe deeper and deeper until you fade off to sleep.

DREAMER'S DELIGHT

When I was younger, I had no problem remembering my dreams. My recall was excellent with plenty of details. As I got older, my dream recall disappeared; I couldn't remember my dreams anymore. It took me years to realize the problem wasn't my recall. The problem was my sleep cycle was so erratic and interrupted, my body wasn't finding the time to dream. I woke up so often, I was never getting into the other stages of sleep.

Now I know how to help my body fall and stay asleep so dreaming can happen.

These herbs help you peacefully sleep and dream. Choose which ones you like and grind together in the ratios you wish with an indica strain.

- Blue vervain
- *Calea zacatechichi*
- Damiana leaf
- Lavender
- Mugwort
- Mullein
- Wild lettuce
- Wormwood

If you are making a tea, experiment with combinations and ratios for your perfect fit and taste preferences. Tinctures can also be combined in different combinations and ratios.

Begin your dream work ritual while you consume your blend, focusing on the words below. If you are not smoking, focus on your "spark" being your initial consumption no matter what method you use:

This spark ignites
My work tonight;
What dreams may come,
Until the sun.

Lie down on your back with your arms comfortably at your sides. Close your eyes and pay attention to your breathing. Focus on holding your tongue at the bottom of your mouth.

As you breathe, think the words:

Show me
What I should see;
Let this weed
Unveil my need.

Begin to slow your breathing until you hit a deep, relaxing pace. Slow the words in time with the slowing of each breath. Remain in the now, focusing on those words as you breathe deeper and deeper. If you have specific dream work to do, set those intentions as you begin to drift off to sleep.

When doing dream work, I have found it beneficial to engage my sense of smell before drifting off to sleep. Incense, an oil diffuser, or aura spray may be helpful for you. The list of herbs for this blend is a great place to start experimenting with incorporating fragrance into your dream work.

DIVINATION

No matter what form of divination you prefer to use—tarot cards, pendulums, scrying mirrors, oracle decks, runes, or others—cannabis and certain herbs can help you connect with the universe, your higher power, or your guides to boost your divination skills and allow you to see and feel answers more clearly.

Choose which ones you like and grind together in the ratios you wish. For this blend you may use either an indica or sativa strain depending on your desires and needs.

- *Calea zacatechichi*
- Mugwort
- Mullein
- Sacred lotus
- White sage
- Wormwood

If you are making a tea, experiment with combinations and ratios for your perfect fit and taste preferences. Tinctures can also be combined in different combinations and ratios.

Set yourself up for your divination session and consume your blend.

Close your eyes and take several deep breaths. Inhale for a count of four; exhale for a count of four. Allow the herbs to work their magic.

Say this either out loud or to yourself as many times as you feel it is necessary; listen to your intuition:

Let this blend
Show the way,
I call these energies
To obey.
Connect me with
My higher power,
My skills to see
Shall be empowered.

When you know you are ready, proceed with your divination. Let the herbs help you do your work.

DRAWING DOWN THE MOON

Drawing down the moon is a phrase used for when a person goes into a trancelike state and invites an aspect of the goddess to join with them, giving the goddess a temporary human vessel. This allows the goddess to speak through a human. The practitioner will also receive an energy surge during the ritual but may feel very drained afterward. It is often performed on the full moon but can be done at other times.

Drawing down the sun is the phrase used when one invites in an aspect of the god, giving him a temporary human vessel. The steps for either are the same, substituting the god for the goddess as presented here. In some traditions, only women may draw down the moon and only men may draw down the sun. As always, you do what works for you. Personally, I don't believe our deities hold our gender against us, and it is important to explore and work with both male and female deities. It is difficult to become at one with the universe if we are avoiding half of it based on gender roles.

For this blend, I recommend using as many of the herbs in the list as possible to boost your power for this working. I always use equal measurements, but you should experiment to find what works best for you.

Combine any of these herbs with either an indica or sativa strain, whichever works best for you.

- Blue vervain
- *Calea zacatechichi*
- Mugwort
- Rose petals
- Sacred lotus
- White sage
- Wormwood

If you are making a tea, experiment with combinations and ratios for your perfect fit and taste preferences. Tinctures can also be combined in different combinations and ratios.

Prepare your ritual location and set up your altar as you normally would. Is there a specific goddess you wish to call upon? Place an icon of her on your altar. Are you seeking connection with an archetype instead of an individual deity? Place items on your altar that represent the archetype. Focus your intention on who you want to connect with as you prepare.

For this type of working, you will want to begin with a protective circle and an opening from your tradition. After your opening, stand or sit (whichever affords you

the most comfort) in the middle of your circle and consume your blend.

Close your eyes and take several deep breaths. Inhale
for a count of four; exhale for a count of four. Allow the
herbs to work their magic.

Focus on who you want to call upon. Open your heart
and your mind. If you feel it, stretch out your arms to
your sides or use them to form a *Y* over your head. Some
call this the "chalice" position and use it when calling to
the goddess. You may also visualize this position as a funnel that helps direct energy into you.

In your mind's eye, reach past your physical environment. Let it all fall away around you. Let everything else
slip away except for your focus on who you wish to bond
with.

Say either to yourself or out loud:

I call to [name or archetype].
I open myself to you,
I offer myself to you
To serve as a vessel
And to become one.

I call to [name or archetype].
I open myself to you,
I offer myself to you
To serve as a vessel
To deliver your wisdom.

I call to [name or archetype].
I open myself to you,
I offer myself to you
To serve as a vessel
To receive your knowledge.
Teach me your way.

When you successfully summon and join with your chosen deity, you will know. There is no doubt in the changes you feel in the energy around you. Pay attention with all your clairsentient abilities. What do you see? What do you hear? What do you feel? Taste? Smell? Each deity has their own distinct aura, meaning each one you work with will present themselves in a different way.

Find the aura with your mind's eye. Direct it toward your "chalice" or "funnel." Absorb the energetic field as it trickles down into you. Feel this new entity as it joins with you. When you feel the shift, lower your arms and close your eyes for a few moments. Allow your connected deity to be the one to reopen them.

It may take several times of trying to be successful. It may also take several successful connections to cope with the awe you may feel. I have occasionally been a bit "starstruck" and too overcome with wonder to go any further with the working. If this happens, know that it will make the next time easier.

Once you have connected with your deity, allow them time to adjust. Let them see your life and events in it through your eyes. Share your joys and sorrows. Give them a taste of what it means to be you. Let them experience you as their vessel, as they allow you to experience them. They have come for a reason. Encourage them, when you are ready, to share their truth with you. What lesson do they have for you? Is there a lesson to be learned? Messages to be passed on to others?

When it is time, you will need to release your deity. To do this, again raise your arms either to your sides or in the form of a *Y* above your head and say:

I release thee, [name or archetype].
I close myself to you.
I have served as your vessel.
Two became one, now one becomes two once more.

I release thee, [name or archetype].
I close myself to you.
I have served as your vessel.
Your wisdom has been received.

I release thee, [name or archetype].
I close myself to you.
I have served as your vessel.
Your way has been learned.

Indulge yourself in a few minutes of relaxing, deep breathing while you come back to yourself alone again. You may feel weak or unsteady. This is normal. It is a good idea to have a grounding yet energizing snack after this working. Cheese and nuts are good options.

Pay attention to how each deity you work with presents themselves to you. Document what your senses tell you in your Book of Shadows or a journal.

As you gain more practice and begin working with different deities, you will be able to recognize who comes to you by the energy they radiate.

When I work with Bloudewedd, she presents as a white and lavender shimmering light. I smell lily of the valley and magnolias—not flowers I would normally associate with her, but they are two of my favorite floral scents. Presenting with scents I know and love is a show of good faith. We are working together. We are combining together. Parts of her, parts of me. I can taste honey on my tongue and hear a soft whispering breeze. I feel younger, more energetic, and sprier. She is the maiden and often invites me to dance.

When I call upon Ganesh, he presents much differently. While the aura around Bloudewedd is light and airy, the one around Ganesh is darker, dustier. The air becomes thick and dry. His arrival is marked with the sounds of heavy breathing. The scent of patchouli is mixed with a musky animal scent. He is the remover of obstacles, and his energy is strong.

Drawing down the moon is an advanced working. If you aren't having any success, that is okay! It will happen for you when you are fully ready. You are experiencing a blockage somewhere. Use your shadow work exercises to see if you can find and overcome the barrier.

———

Blends draw upon new energies for your magical workings to enhance your experience. There are endless possibilities to the blends you can concoct for your practice. In our next chapter, we will work with blends that help enhance the energies present in the cycle of the year.

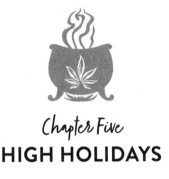

Chapter Five
HIGH HOLIDAYS

I will be the first to admit, I can find any reason to have a party. And why not? Parties are great fun: people laughing, talking, dancing, drumming, and singing, and kids running around and playing. We enjoy them because they are an extended act of positive energy raising. They give us a boost and send goodness into the universe. The positive energy raised at a party or other special event can affect the participants for days and even in memories for years to come. At The Gathering Grove, we hold family-friendly rituals at each of the sabbats, outdoors when we can. These festivals are effective in recharging, refreshing, and rejuvenating the participants with the energies we raise.

No matter what your tradition is, participating in rituals for sabbats and moons is a way of raising energy and working with the natural energies of the year. Each of the sabbats is connected to a specific high energy point of the year or to the liminal times between. Ostara is the vernal equinox and the beginning of astronomical spring. Midsummer is the summer solstice and the beginning of summer. Mabon, or the autumnal equinox, begins fall, and Yule with the winter solstice is the beginning of winter. Imbolg, Beltane, Lughnasadh, and Samhain take place about halfway into each season. They are the liminal times when we see the end of one season and the beginning of the next.

Working with cannabis is another way in which we work in a liminal time. When we hit a peak experience, we are not fully here nor there, but in between. One of the characteristics of a peak experience is the slowing of time. When your experience is over, you may have felt like an hour has gone by only to be surprised to find it's only been twenty minutes.

In these rituals, we will employ the energies of the year, along with appropriate blends to boost our magical workings. Each ritual is presented in its most elaborate form with several supplies. Eliminate what you wish for a simpler practice.

IMBOLG

Imbolg is the first sabbat of the calendar year. It is also the first of the sabbats that falls during a liminal time. Winter begins with Yule on December 21, and spring begins on the vernal equinox, with Imbolg falling about halfway between the two. Also known as Candlemas, St. Brighid's Day, and even Groundhog's Day, it is celebrated as the time when the earth begins stirring to awaken from its deep winter slumber.

While spring may be on the way, certain areas definitely do not feel like it. Where I live in northern Illinois, we see the worst of winter in February. We have our coldest temperatures, and the majority of our snow falls then. It doesn't feel like it's almost spring. Even when it's spring here, it often doesn't feel like spring. This year we had a seventy-one-degree day in winter and then followed it up a month later with an inch of snow on April 2. We have been known to get snow as late as halfway through May.

In other parts of the world, where the change of seasons isn't as noticeable, these liminal periods blend and hide. They are there but are more difficult to be seen when looking into the natural world around us.

This liminal time can feel unsettling. As this transition takes place, energies shift back and forth between the two sides. Imbolg is a time you may feel yourself still being pulled to rest as in winter while also being pushed to spring forward into action. Cabin fever often hits at this time of year for those of us in cooler regions. We are told the earth is awakening, we are told it is time to turn our focus from inner workings to outer workings, but when we can't see or feel those changes in the environment, it may make it more difficult to feel and initiate those changes in ourselves. Additionally, we have become accustomed to instant gratification. These stretched-out, variable energies of nature go against what society has taught us is "natural," which is why we may feel unsettled or confused.

In this ritual, we will open ourselves to recognize, experience, and accept the differences of these energies. Even if you are adept at singling them out and working with them already, this ritual allows you to celebrate this time between.

For this ritual you will need:

- Representations of earth (salt, eggshells, or dirt), fire (candle), water (moon water), and air (incense or a feather)
- Lighter
- Ground cannabis (indica) to mix with the following in a blend:
  - Dried and crushed, or ground cloves (a little goes a long way)

– Dried crushed mugwort

(This blend may also be made as a tea or in tinctures; prepare what you need ahead of time. If you are making a tea, you will need to have a pot of hot water and cup. If there isn't room for these on your altar, it is okay to leave them off, but place them close by.)

• Mortar and pestle

• Small spoon

• Small decorative container for your blend (You will make the blend as a part of the ritual.)

• Your ritual smoking piece, or supplies for your preferred method of consuming cannabis

• Comfortable way to sit on the ground, such as a meditation cushion or pillow

• A white chime candle or spell size candle with holder

Optional:
• Deity statues

• Any other altar decorations you would like to include

Set up your altar, leaving space in the center for your smoking piece or supplies needed for your preferred consumption method, cannabis, and ground cloves and mugwort along with a small empty container or bowl in which to mix your blend. After you grind each herb, empty the mortar into your chosen container. Once they are all ground, you can either blend them together in the mortar or the container, whichever allows you the room to do so. If you are using tinctures, mix those together in your decorative container. You will want to be about eye level with the white candle, which should also be placed near the center of your altar.

You may use your own opening or the one included here.

Light your incense representing air and wave it around, allowing the smoke to whirl and swirl around you. If you are using a feather instead, wave it around in the air. Say:

> *I call upon the air,*
> *Guardian of intuition.*
> *Join with me in this rite*
> *To guide me along my path.*

Light the candle representing fire and say:

> *I call upon the fire,*
> *Guardian of self-knowledge.*
> *Join with me in this rite*
> *To guide me along my path.*

Pour the moon water in a circle around your altar and sacred space and say:

> I call upon the water,
> Guardian of emotions.
> Join with me in this rite
> To guide me along my path.

If you are using salt or dirt for earth and can sprinkle it on the ground around your altar and sacred space, do so. Say:

> I call upon the earth,
> Guardian of stability.
> Join with me in this rite
> To guide me along my path.

Take a moment to center and direct your focus. Invite your deity or deities to join with you or call upon your higher self by saying:

> I call upon [name or archetype],
> To learn from and to commune with.
> Join with me in this rite
> And guide me on my path.

Pause for a moment to refocus your mind on your next task: combining and mixing your blend together in the mortar and pestle.

Add a small amount of ground clove into the mortar. Say:

> *May this clove raise my awareness*
> *To the energies around me,*
> *Both seen and unseen.*

Add a small spoonful of the mugwort into the mortar and say:

> *May this mugwort ferry me through this liminal realm.*

If you are using tinctures, add as many drops of each to your container to blend.

Add as much cannabis as you like into the mortar and begin grinding and blending. As you work, say:

> *Guide me on this journey,*
> *With this blend I make.*
> *Guide me on this journey,*
> *I now prepare to take.*

Add your cannabis blend to your sacred piece, or prepare your tea or tincture. Seat yourself in a comfortable position to consume your blend (with refills as necessary) where you will be able to see the flame of the white candle once it is lit.

Once you feel centered and focused, consume your blend and close your eyes for a moment. Slow your breathing. Inhale for a count of five, hold for a count of five, exhale for a count of five. Feel the energies of the herbs in your system. Consume more if needed.

When you feel relaxed and at ease, reopen your eyes and light your candle. Say:

> *As I light this flame,*
> *I focus on the light.*

Stare into the flame. Focus on the flickering. Notice how it moves back and forth. The flame may grow and shrink, move left and right. The intensity of the flame fluctuates but still burns the candle. It still serves its purpose— it gives light, it gives warmth. You can see the changes as they occur.

Depending on your abilities, you may be able to feel these fluctuations as they occur too. Practice feeling these changes by reaching out with your own energies to connect with them.

Like the flame of the candle, the energies at this time of the year fluctuate. Some of these energies you can see or feel the effects of: the warmth of the sun on the ground or the brisk slap of a strong north wind. Other energies you may not see but you might still feel: The push and pull between the seasons. The push and pull between inner workings and outer workings. The push and pull between rest and action.

Once you have concentrated on the flame for several minutes, you may either let it continue to burn if it is safe or go ahead and extinguish it. Consume more of your blend. You want to be able to hit a peak experience if possible.

Close your eyes. Relax.

Allow the mundane world to fall away. Let the walls that surround you dissolve. Connect with your higher self. Call to your deity if you desire. Let the connection occur in whatever way it needs to. Allow yourself to be led and guided instead of fighting to follow your own way. Feel yourself at one with the universe. When you are there, you will know.

Ask the universe to show you these energies associated with this time of year. They may appear to you in any of many different ways. You may see colors, shapes, waves, or symbols that represent them. Ask the universe to show you the differences so you may better recognize and distinguish them from one another.

Feel the push and pull of each of these energies. Experience how they purposely keep change happening at a slow pace. There is a shift, ever so slight, that works to form the circular pattern of a year.

The universe will explain and teach you if you let it. Listen to what it tells you. There is a lesson for you if you but listen.

Recognize what is good in each of these energies, what is important. What joy can they bring you? How do they help you? Do you feel a push or pull to shift your own energies from internal to external before the natural world around you is doing the same? Do you find it difficult to reengage after a season of rest?

Ask the universe to guide you in the areas you need help adjusting. Listen to the messages the universe has for you; it will let you know where both your strengths and your weaknesses lie. It will gently teach you how to work with these fluctuating energies.

When it is time for your peak to end, it will.

Take a moment to center and redirect your focus.

Release your deity or deities by saying:

> *I thank you, [name or archetype],*
> *Your presence in this rite*
> *Guides me on my path.*

Release each of the elements, saying:

> *I thank the air,*
> *Guardian of intuition.*
> *Your presence in this rite*
> *Guides me on my path.*

I thank the fire,
Guardian of self-knowledge.
Your presence in this rite
Guides me on my path.

I thank the water,
Guardian of emotions.
Your presence in this rite
Guides me on my path.

I thank the earth,
Guardian of stability.
Your presence in this rite
Guides me on my path.

If you like, you may close your ritual with a statement such as "So mote it be" or "My circle is open but unbroken."

Instead of finding these energies confusing or trying to fight them, we must remind ourselves, nature takes her time when she wants to. She doesn't make the switch from winter to spring overnight. The shift in energies is gradual. It takes weeks. There is no instant gratification. Instead of wanting spring to quickly take over, we need to learn the patience to wait it out. Mother Nature takes her time to wake up; who are we to tell her she is doing it wrong? It is not Mother Nature who needs to speed up; it is humans who need to learn to slow down. Following the energies of nature instead of trying to speed them up or fighting against them teaches us patience and reminds us rest is a necessity, not a luxury.

OSTARA / VERNAL EQUINOX

Ostara, also known as the vernal or spring equinox, is a time of both balance and new beginnings. It is the official start of spring. For those who live in a four seasons climate, it is the time when the snow melts away while new life bursts through the thawing ground. Day and night are relatively equal, and after today, the light will reign until the autumnal equinox when darkness wins out once again. We turn our focus from inner workings to outer workings. Like the buds on the leaves, we are ready to burst forth with new energy to experience fresh growth.

In this ritual, we will celebrate the rebirth of spring and the world around us while working with the natural energies of the year to progress in our practice. Since the spring is a time of rebirth and planting seeds, this is where we will focus. We will perform a meditation with a custom smoke blend to connect with our higher selves (or other higher power). This meditation will help us to look at what we need and what changes we must make to give ourselves a new start in whatever area of our lives we want to improve. What goals do we want to set? What seeds do we want to plant and watch grow to maturity in our lives? What do we wish to harvest? Your answers can be related to either your spiritual practice or goals in the mundane world.

After the meditation, we will plant those seeds along with flower seeds (or herbs—something suitable for the container you choose to use) to tend to as we work toward the goals we want to achieve.

Read through the entire ritual first, particularly the meditation, to better guide yourself along.

For this ritual you will need:

- Comfortable way to sit on the ground, such as a meditation cushion or pillow
- Representations of earth, fire, water, and incense for air—make them fitting for the occasion:
  - A bowl of dirt, salt, or crushed eggshells for earth
  - An egg-shaped candle for fire
  - A pastel-colored glass bottle or pitcher filled with moon water
  - Incense with the scent of spring flowers
- Lighter
- Chime or spell size candles with holders. You will need one blue, one yellow, one pink, and one green.

- Ground cannabis (indica suggested; however, you may also try this with a sativa) to mix with the following herbs in a blend:
    - Dried crushed violets
    - Dried crushed blue lotus flower petals
    - Dried crushed rose petals
    - Dried crushed mugwort

    (This blend may also be made as a tea or in tinctures; prepare what you need ahead of time. If you are making a tea, you will need to have a pot of hot water and cup. If there isn't room for these on your altar, it is okay to leave them off, but place them close by.)

- Mortar and pestle
- A spoon
- Small decorative container for your blend (You will make the blend as a part of the ritual.)
- Your ritual smoking piece, or supplies for your preferred method of consuming cannabis
- Strips of paper, any length about an inch wide
- Pen
- A planter filled with potting soil
- Flower or herb seeds

Optional:

- Any spring-themed decorations you would like to include

- Any deity statues you would like to include

If it's possible, perform this ritual outside. For those who have been cooped up with cold weather, Ostara may be your first chance of the year to perform an outdoor ritual. Place your meditation cushion or pillow in front of the altar on the ground. You may begin the ritual standing and wait until your meditation to sit if it is easier for you. If getting up and down is an issue, you may sit in a comfortable chair; otherwise, try to keep as much connection to the ground as possible. You may also set up your altar directly on the ground.

When setting your altar, be sure the candles are in safe holders and not in danger of catching anything on fire around you while you meditate.

You may use your own opening or the one included here.

Light your incense representing air and wave it around, allowing the smoke to whirl and swirl around you, or waft your feather and say:

I call upon the air,
Bringer of intuition.

Join with me in ritual
And guide me on my path.

Light the candle representing fire and say:

I call upon the fire,
Bringer of self-knowledge.
Join with me in ritual
And guide me on my path.

Pour the moon water in a circle around your altar and sacred space and say:

I call upon the water,
Bringer of emotions.
Join with me in ritual
And guide me on my path.

If you are using salt or dirt for earth and can sprinkle it on the ground around your altar and sacred space, do so. Say:

I call upon the earth,
Bringer of stability.
Join with me in ritual
And guide me on my path.

Take a moment to center and direct your focus. Invite your deity or deities to join with you or call upon your higher self by saying:

> I call upon [name or archetype],
> Bringer(s) of wisdom.
> Join with me in ritual
> And guide me on my path.

Light the blue candle and say:

> Bring to me calmness and tranquility,
> Grant me patience and comprehension.

Light the yellow candle and say:

> Aid my communication and intuition,
> Grant me joy and vitality.

Light the pink candle and say:

> Aid me in my spiritual healing,
> Grant me contentment and harmony.

Light the green candle and say:

> Aid me in my new beginnings,
> Grant me growth and abundance.

Pause for a moment to refocus your mind on your next task: combining and mixing your blend together in the mortar and pestle. After you grind each herb, empty the mortar into your chosen container. Once they are all ground, you can either blend them together in the mortar or the container, whichever allows you the room to do so. If you are using tinctures, add as many drops of each one you want into your container to blend. Add a small spoonful of the violets into the mortar. Say:

Guide me in my spiritual healing,
Grant my wish to bring me balance.

Add a small spoonful of the blue lotus flower petals into the mortar and say:

Guide me on my journey,
Grant me peace along the way.

Add a small spoonful of the rose petals into the mortar and say:

Protect me on my journey,
Increase my psychic energies.

Add a small spoonful of the mugwort into the mortar and say:

> *Guide me on my journey,*
> *Take me where I need to go.*

Add as much cannabis as you like into the mortar and begin grinding and blending. As you work, say:

> *Guide me on this journey,*
> *With this blend I make.*
> *Guide me on this journey,*
> *I now prepare to take.*

Add your cannabis blend to your sacred piece, or prepare your preferred method of consuming cannabis. Seat yourself in a comfortable position to take your blend (with as many refills as necessary) and perform the following meditation.

> *Slow your breathing. Inhale for a count of five, hold for a count of five, exhale for a count of five. Take a moment to relax, ground, and center. Feel the energies of the herbs in your system.*
>
> *Allow the mundane world to fall completely away. Let any walls that surround you drop away. Connect with your higher self. Feel yourself at one with the universe. Call to your deity if you desire.*
>
> *At Ostara, you look to bring balance into your life. Balance between work and play. Balance*

between activity and rest. Balance in your relation-
ships with equal amounts of give and take. Stabil-
ity. Equity. Harmony.

How can you bring these qualities out in your
life? Focus on the steps you need to make to intro-
duce, increase, or accentuate balance in your life.
What first steps must you take to achieve these
goals?

What other goals do you want to set for your-
self? What harvest do you want to reap? Listen to
what your higher voice or power says to you. Let
them guide you to what you need.

When you have the answers you are looking for, open
your eyes, and using the strips of paper and the pen, sum
up your goals and write them down in brief sentences or
keywords correlating to your future steps. You may stand
and stretch whenever needed.

Roll each strip of paper tightly into a tiny tube and
push completely into the dirt of the planter around the
outside edge. Do this for each piece of paper. As you roll
and push each one in, say:

This seed I plant
To tend and grow,
Calls forth a future
I wish to know.

Sprinkle the flower or herbal seeds you are planting over the top and gently use a spoon to cover them. Say:

> As these seeds
> Sprout and grow,
> So does the future
> I work to know.

Water the seeds with your moon water and say:

> This water blessed
> By the light of the moon,
> Helps the seed and soil
> To commune.
>
> Its energy
> Helps the two combine,
> Becoming one
> To grow and thrive.
>
> These seeds I plant,
> Along with mine,
> My goals achieved
> Is what I strive.

Envision what the future looks like with your goals accomplished. See everything as you wish for it to be. Your goals accomplished, dreams fulfilled. Experience the feelings of satisfaction and courage, and take pride in

your achievements. Pour the energies from these emotions into your planter, same as you did with your moon
water. Feel the energies build up inside you, travel down
your arm, into your hand, and spill out as you tip your
hand over the planter. "Water" your seeds with this
energy. Your intuition will tell you when your "watering"
is complete.

Take a moment to center and redirect your focus.
Release your deity or deities by saying:

> I thank you, [name or archetype],
> Bringer(s) of wisdom.
> Your presence in this ritual
> Guides me on my path.

Release each of the elements, saying:

> I thank the air,
> Bringer of intuition.
> Your presence in this ritual
> Guides me on my path.

> I thank the fire,
> Bringer of self-knowledge.
> Your presence in this ritual
> Guides me on my path.

I thank the water,
Bringer of emotions.
Your presence in this ritual
Guides me on my path.

I thank the earth,
Bringer of stability.
Your presence in this ritual
Guides me on my path.

Keep your planter in a place where it will receive regular sunlight, and water it as needed. Water the goals you planted by working toward them in the mundane world. Let your plant and goals grow together. Your plant serves as a reminder that mundane work and spellwork must always go hand in hand. Energy from two realms is more powerful than energy from only one.

BELTANE

Beltane is the halfway point between Ostara and Midsummer and known as a fire and fertility festival. It is again a liminal time, halfway between the beginning of spring and the beginning of summer.

The grass has turned green, and flowers are starting to bloom. The world feels alive again. The darkness of winter is gone. The barren trees have been overrun with buds bursting, unfurling newborn leaves.

The energy surge is undeniable. There is excitement. There is life. A primal desire floats in the spiritual sphere. The new life in nature breathes new life into us. We feel refreshed. We feel fertile—not necessarily only in a sexual or reproductive sense, but in other productive ways. All the energy we have stored up during the resting months is pouring forth. Our plans are being put into action. Goals are being worked on and completed. The sun sets later, giving us the illusion of longer days. We can feel the energy all around us. We can connect with it, especially in a natural setting. We can share and exchange energies with this life force, and because Beltane falls at an in-between time, it also possesses its own liminal magic to assist in the connection with the energies of the natural world.

The most optimal times to perform this ritual would be sunset on April 30, midnight of April 30, or sunrise on May 1: times of a liminal nature. These times are not required, only optimal.

You will need a location where it is safe to move around and dance; outside is best if possible. Substitute an open window if you must. If you have access to a firepit, bonfire, or outdoor fireplace, build a fire with Mary Jane magical mulch and cannabis kindling as your fire base for this working. (If you have them!) Again, ensure you have plenty of room for safety. Remember, you can also build a small fire in a cauldron if you do not have access to a firepit. If you need to perform the ritual indoors, use a tea light candle set into a bowl of sand to represent your Beltane fire.

Since we will be working with music for this ritual, you will need a playlist. (At the end of the book, you can find info to check out the Spotify lists we use.) How long you make your playlist is entirely up to you. I recommend beginning with a slower song, progressing through faster music to build and release energy, followed by a cooldown. You can repeat this cycle as many times as you want. You know what your physical capabilities and limitations are, so do what works for you. For those with mobility issues, dancing does not have to require you being on your feet. Try sitting in a chair and moving your body in different ways to the music. Dance is not only a specific set of choreographed steps. In fact, I discourage it. Move your body in ways that make it feel good. That is the only requirement you need to meet, especially for your personal spiritual workings. Stretch out muscles you seldom use. Rotate joints. Feel the rhythm in your body and the music in your soul. Let your body move the way it wants to.

Look for music that emphasizes and represents the theme "primal nature." This can be through lyrics or through the notes and instruments. What songs fill your body, mind, and soul with passion, lust, and a zest for life? Throw them on your playlist. Beltane is the perfect time to connect with your primal instinctual nature; it has much to teach you about life and letting go of unimportant things.

For this ritual you will need:

- You may use a table or other surface for an altar or set it up directly on the ground
- Representations of earth (salt, eggshells, or dirt), fire (bonfire, cauldron fire, or a tea light), water (moon water), and air (incense or a feather)
- Lighter
- Ground cannabis (sativa) to mix with the following in a blend:
  - Dried crushed hop flowers
  - Dried crushed wormwood
  - Dried crushed California poppy
  - Dried crushed rose petals
  - Dried crushed damiana leaf

– Dried crushed blue lotus flower

– Dried crushed mugwort

(This blend may also be made as a tea or in tinctures; prepare what you need ahead of time. If you are making a tea, you will need to have a pot of hot water and cup. If there isn't room for these on your altar, it is okay to leave them off, but place them close by.)

- Mortar and pestle
- Small spoon
- Small decorative container for your blend (You will make the blend as a part of the ritual.)
- Your ritual smoking piece, or supplies for your preferred method of consuming cannabis
- Dress in loose, comfortable clothing
- Music and a way to play it
- A healthy grounding snack or meal

Optional:
- If you like, have a sativa vape on hand for boosting along with your blend
- Mary Jane magical mulch
- Cannabis kindling
- Any deity statues you would like to include
- Fresh flowers are a perfect altar decoration for Beltane

- If you are able to perform this ritual outdoors, consider having a blanket or chair available for rest breaks

Light your bonfire, cauldron fire, or tea light in sand to represent fire. Proceed with your own opening or the one included here.

Light your incense representing air and wave it around, allowing the smoke to whirl and swirl, or waft a feather in the air around you. Say:

> I invite the guardian of air,
> Let the winds of intuition blow.
> Join with me in this rite
> And guide me on my path.

Light the candle representing fire and say:

> I invite the guardian of fire,
> Let the flames of knowledge burn.
> Join with me in this rite
> And guide me on my path.

Pour the moon water in a circle around your altar and sacred space and say:

> I invite the guardian of water,
> Let the waves of emotions flow.

Join with me in this rite
And guide me on my path.

If you are using salt or dirt for earth and can sprinkle it on the ground around your altar and sacred space, do so. Say:

I invite the guardian of earth,
Be my grounding rock of stability.
Join with me in this rite
And guide me on my path.

Take a moment to center and direct your focus. Invite your deity or deities to join with you or call upon your higher self by saying:

I call upon [name or archetype],
To learn from and to commune with.
Join with me in this rite
And guide me on my path.

Pause for a moment to refocus your mind on your next task: combining and mixing your blend together in the mortar and pestle.

Pour a small amount of each of the herbs and flowers to grind together into your blend. If you are using tinctures, add as many drops of each to your container to blend.

Mugwort can be difficult to work with, so feel free to rip it apart with your fingers if needed to ensure it gets blended together. (I use about a tablespoon of each; for things like flower petals, which will break down much smaller than their original size, I use a heaping tablespoon. For herbs that are already dried and crushed, I will use more of an unpacked, level tablespoon.)

Add as much cannabis as you like into the mortar and begin grinding and blending. As you work, say:

> *Guide me on this journey,*
> *With this blend I make.*
> *Guide me on this journey,*
> *I now prepare to take.*

While you blend these together, think about the previously discussed qualities: primal, lustful, passionate, energetic, fiery. These herbs, especially when combined with cannabis, will help raise these feelings in you. These energies are your focus.

Add your Beltane blend to your sacred piece, or prepare your preferred method of consumption. Seat yourself in a comfortable position to take your blend (with as many refills as necessary). You may want to set up your playlist to have a slower song play while you center your thoughts and experience your blend. Remember, when smoking blends, it will generally cut down on the amount of cannabis you are smoking. It's okay to smoke several bowls or refill a bong several times to give your body, mind, and spirit enough THC to get them to where they need to go.

Give yourself time to start feeling the effects. Let your body move to the music as you load up on your blend. Feel the walls coming down around you. Allow yourself to connect with spirit.

When you are ready, get yourself up from your seated position and start moving. Feel the music in your body and spirit and let yourself move in whatever ways feel good. If it's safe to do so (far enough away from lit candles, fire, or other obstacles), close your eyes and raise your face to the sky. This helps you let go and slip into the time between time, the liminal zone where a peak experience makes the mundane world fade and the spiritual realm claims dominance.

Dance throughout your playlist. Experiment expressing with your movements and motions the energetic qualities you have been focusing on. Let your body, mind, and spirit all experience them.

Does your deity or higher self have a message or lesson for you while you experience these energies? Ask. There is always more to learn. Let your spirit be guided through dance and thought.

Twirl and whirl, stomp, kick, snake your arms and torso. Let your body move in ways it doesn't normally move. Our brains tell our bodies how to move; let your spirit tell your body how to move instead. Let your spirit express passion. Let your spirit express lust. Let your spirit express its own primal needs.

Focus your intention on accomplishing the goals you previously set. Focus on manifesting what it is you desire to bring into your life.

Release your built-up energy, sending your intention out into the universe. When you release, do so vocally too. There are many ways to vocally release energy, from yells and whoops to howls and growls. Do what feels right for you.

Rebuild the energy again if you planned it with your playlist. After your final energy release, tumble to the earth or gently slide back into your chair. A blanket can deal with dew-covered grass; however, rolling in the damp coolness can also be quite refreshing after raising your heartbeat in dance.

Enjoy and express the exhilaration.

Relax and give your heart rate time to slow to normal once again. Slip from the ethereal realm back into the realm of the mundane. Ground. Feel the solid, stable earth below you. Let any excess energy drip from you in rivulets and run off to the ground.

Breathe deeply with your eyes closed.

When you are ready, take a moment to center and re-direct your focus. Either remain in position or stand.

Release your deity or deities by saying:

> *I thank you, [name or archetype].*
> *Your presence in my rites*
> *Helps to guide me on my path.*

Release each of the elements, saying:

> *I thank the guardian of air.*
> *Your presence in my rites*
> *Helps to guide me on my path.*

> *I thank the guardian of fire.*
> *Your presence in my rites*
> *Helps to guide me on my path.*

> *I thank the guardian of water.*
> *Your presence in my rites*
> *Helps to guide me on my path.*

> *I thank the guardian of earth.*
> *Your presence in my rites*
> *Helps to guide me on my path.*

> *My rite is over.*
> *My circle is open.*

Replenish and ground yourself after this rite with a healthy snack: seeds, nuts, berries, cheese, and cut raw veggies are all excellent options (especially combined), and drink plenty of water. Infused waters add to both the taste and your grounding experience. Water can be infused with a variety of herbs, fruits, and vegetables. Cucumber mint water is refreshing, while a watermelon basil may be less stimulating. Try to use what is locally in season.

Experienced practitioners may want to begin this ritual with a drawing down of the moon or sun ritual or enjoy part of the dance themselves before adding in the drawing down ritual. Do what works for you.

Where there is enough space, this rite can easily be adapted to a group ritual.

MIDSUMMER

Though we call it Midsummer, it truly is only the beginning of astronomical summer. It is also the day with (technically) the longest amount of daylight of the year, with the veil between the human world and the realm of the Fae at its thinnest. The natural world is in full bloom. Gardens, vines, and other plants have begun bearing fruit. Birds and animals have hatched or birthed their young. The energies present currently focus primarily on growth and abundance. The powerful force of life is all around you and can be tapped into—if you know how to recognize it and connect with it.

At Beltane, the strongest energies we focused on were passion, lust, fire, and our own primal natures. These energies continue throughout the light half of the year; however, as the year evolves, the most abundant energies shift. We turn our focus now to growth, strength, and abundance as the dominant energies.

This ritual will focus on connecting with this life force, replenishing yourself, and sending this energy toward your manifestations. We will once again be using dance (like for Beltane) but with a different tempo, a new blend, and fresh intentions.

The most optimal times to perform this ritual would be sunset on Midsummer eve, midnight of Midsummer eve, or sunrise on Midsummer day. These times are not required, only optimal.

You will need a safe place for this ritual, preferably outdoors in an area where you can connect with the energies from nature and the local wildlife. Substitute an open window if you must. Add a live plant to your window ledge or altar if you need to be indoors to help boost the connection to the energies of the world outside.

If you have access to a firepit, bonfire, or outdoor fireplace, use it. Prepare your fire with Mary Jane magical mulch and cannabis kindling if you have them. Always ensure you have plenty of room for safety. You can build a small fire in a cauldron if you do not have access to a firepit. If you need to perform the ritual indoors, use a tea light candle set into a bowl of sand to represent your fire.

Instead of fast, upbeat music, your playlist should be of a slower, mystical, more ethereal nature. Think about what you want to connect with: the energy of the life force of the trees, grass, flowers, birds, and animals around you. What type of music do you think will help you make this connection? You will be working on replenishing your own energy and sending energy to what you are working on manifesting in your life. You will still want to put your slowest songs first and last, with faster songs in the middle, but you do not want to wear yourself out. Instead, you will be focusing on absorbing the robust and potent energies brimming with life to revive and replenish your own energy. Make your playlist whatever length you prefer.

The same energies we will be working with are energies also used by and connected to the Fae, as they are a part of the plant spirit world. It is no coincidence that when nature is at its strongest and fullest part of the growth cycle, that is also when the veil between the human world and the realm of the Fae is the thinnest. When you are done with your dance, leave an offering of milk and honey.

Let them know the space is now available for their use, pre-energized.

For this ritual you will need:

- You may use a table or other surface for an altar or set it up directly on the ground
- Representations of earth (salt, eggshells, or dirt), fire (candle or torch), water (moon water), and air (incense or a feather)
- Lighter
- Ground cannabis (indica) to mix with the following in a blend:
    - Dried crushed lavender
    - Dried crushed hop flowers
    - Dried crushed wormwood
    - Dried crushed rose petals
    - Dried crushed damiana leaf
    - Dried crushed blue lotus flower
    - Dried crushed mugwort

        (This blend may also be made as a tea or in tinctures; prepare what you need ahead of time. If you are making a tea, you will need to have a pot of hot water and cup. If there isn't room for these on your altar, it is okay to leave them off, but place them close by.)

- Mortar and pestle

- Small spoon
- Small decorative container for your blend (You will make the blend as a part of the ritual.)
- Your ritual smoking piece, or supplies for your preferred method of consuming cannabis
- Music and a way to play it
- Dress in loose, comfortable, lightweight clothing that reveals as much skin as you are comfortable with
- A healthy grounding snack or meal

Optional:
- Mary Jane magical mulch
- Cannabis kindling
- If you like, have an indica vape on hand for boosting along with your blend.
- Any deity statues and altar decorations you would like to include
- Offerings for the Fae
- If indoors, a plant to help with the connection
- If you perform this ritual outdoors, consider having a blanket or chair available for rest breaks.

Light your bonfire, cauldron fire, or tea light in sand to represent fire. Proceed with your own opening or the one included here.

Light your incense representing air and wave it around, allowing the smoke to whirl and swirl, or waft a feather in the air around you. Say:

> *I call upon the spirit of air,*
> *Let your winds of intuition blow.*
> *Join with me in this rite*
> *To guide me on my path.*

Light the candle representing fire and say:

> *I call upon the spirit of fire,*
> *Let your flames of knowledge burn.*
> *Join with me in this rite*
> *To guide me on my path.*

Pour the moon water in a circle around your altar and sacred space and say:

> *I call upon the spirit of water,*
> *Let your waves of emotions flow.*
> *Join with me in this rite*
> *To guide me on my path.*

If you are using salt or dirt for earth and can sprinkle it on the ground around your altar and sacred space, do so. Say:

I call upon the spirit of earth,
Let your base of stability ground me.
Join with me in this rite
To guide me on my path.

Take a moment to center and direct your focus. Invite your deity or deities to join with you or call upon your higher self by saying:

I call upon [name or archetype],
Join with me in this rite
To guide me on my path.

Pause for a moment to refocus your mind on preparing your blend.

Pour a small amount of each of the herbs and flowers to grind together into your blend. After you grind each herb, empty the mortar into your chosen container. Once they are all ground, you can either blend them together in the mortar or the container, whichever allows you the room to do so. If you are using tinctures, add as many drops of each as you want to your container to blend.

Mugwort can be difficult to work with, so feel free to rip it apart with your fingers if needed to ensure it gets blended together. (I use about a tablespoon of each; things like flower petals, which will break down much smaller than their original size, I use a heaping tablespoon. For herbs that are already dried and crushed, I will use more of an unpacked, level tablespoon.)

Add as much cannabis as you like into the mortar and begin grinding and blending. As you work, say:

> *Guide me on this journey,*
> *With this blend I make.*
> *Guide me on this journey,*
> *I now prepare to take.*

While you blend these together, think about the previously discussed qualities: growth, strength, and abundance. These energies are your focus. For this working you will want to draw from these energies in the environment around you, infuse them with the goals you want to manifest, and then release them back into the universe, sending your manifestations with them—sort of like responding to an incoming email and attaching a file along with your reply.

Add your Midsummer blend to your sacred piece, or prepare your preferred method of consuming cannabis. Seat yourself in a comfortable position to consume your blend (with as many refills as necessary). Remember, when working with blends, it will cut down on the amount of cannabis you intake at a time, so be sure to make up for it by smoking more.

Give yourself time to start feeling the effects. Let your body move to the music as you load up on your blend. Feel the walls coming down around you. Allow yourself to connect with spirit.

When you are ready, get yourself up from your seated position and start moving. Feel the music in your body and spirit and let yourself move in whatever ways feel good. Express yourself. If it's safe to do so (far enough away from lit candles, fire, or other obstacles), close your eyes and raise your face to the sky to help slip into a peak experience and the spiritual realm.

Keep your movements toned down to a comfortable, slow pace. No need to work up a sweat. Instead of raising energy, you will be acquiring it, infusing it, and releasing it.

Some people will be able to see the different energies on their own—the different life forces from flora and fauna, along with the energies that propel them to grow and prosper. It can take years of practice, but learning to sense and distinguish the energies around you is an excellent skill to perfect.

If you cannot see these energies already, the first step is to open your mind and pretend you do. What do you think they would look like? Imagine what it would be like to see the auras of each and every living organism around you.

Think of what it looks like when a clap of dust hits a sunbeam. All the little particles floating by, dancing through the light. Put your arms out to your sides and let them stretch and sway back and forth several times. Move them over your head and again back and forth from left to right, stirring up the air around you. Visualize the energies swirling together all around you like the dust in the sunbeam. Float away in the dance with them.

Enjoy the experience. No expectations, simply letting your mind float around with the different energies while your body gently stirs them up.

When you are ready to move on, pause your dance (not your music) and put your skin to work. Skin is the largest organ in your body, and it is an excellent conductor and detector of electricity and other types of energies. Think of the goosebumps you get when you hear an excellent singer or if a lightning strike occurs close by; both are types of energy you can detect through your skin.

If you are already adept at distinguishing and siphoning energies, go ahead and extract the ones we are looking for.

For those who need practice, find the energies you are looking for in your "sunbeam" visualization. Attempt distinguishing the energies from one another. What makes them different? What do they look like? What do they feel like when they trace along your skin? Slowly wave your arms around in your "sunbeam" and collect the energies you are seeking on your skin. Feel these energies gently piercing through your skin and into your soul as you confidently perform your harvest.

Talk to these energies as they swirl, snake, and surge throughout your body and spirit. Infuse them with your plans, your wishes, your desires, your wants, and needs. All that you want to manifest, pour into these newly gathered energy waves.

To release these energies, take deep breaths, filling your lungs and channeling the now-infused energies into the air in your lungs. Exhale with a deep, strong *whoooooosh* through your lips. Continue the cycle as long as you want—absorbing the energy through your skin, infusing it with your manifestation intentions, and releasing it back into the universe through your breath.

When you are finished, gently fall to the ground or slide back into your chair. Slip from the ethereal realm back to the world of the mundane. Ground. Feel the solid, stable earth below you. Let any excess energy evaporate into the air around you.

Breathe deeply with your eyes closed.

Take a moment to center and redirect your focus. Either remain in position or stand.

Release your deity or deities by saying:

I thank you, [name or archetype].
Your presence in my rites
Helps to guide me on my path.

Release each of the elements, saying:

I thank the spirit of air.
Your presence in my rites
Guides me on my path.

I thank the spirit of fire.
Your presence in my rites
Guides me on my path.

I thank the spirit of water.
Your presence in my rites
Guides me on my path.

I thank the spirit of earth.
Your presence in my rites
Guides me on my path.

Replenish and ground yourself after this rite with a healthy, locally in season snack and suitably infused water.

Experienced practitioners may want to begin this ritual with a drawing down of the moon or sun ritual or enjoy part of the dance themselves before adding in the drawing down ritual. Do what works for you.

Where there is enough space, this rite can easily be adapted to a group ritual.

LUGHNASADH/LAMMAS

Whether you refer to this holiday as Lughnasadh or as Lammas, it is the first harvest festival of the year and is generally observed on August 1 or at sunset on July 31. This is when we begin to harvest the first goods from our gardens. Traditionally, this day is celebrated with the baking of bread.

It is also when we begin to harvest some of the short-term goals we set for ourselves back in the spring. It's time to evaluate and see which goals have been completed, which need more attention, which are close to completion and need finishing up, which ones may need some revamping, or which ones have completely stalled out.

As the halfway point between astronomical summer and astronomical fall, we again find ourselves in a liminal period, making this an ideal time to take a moment to review the progress you have made and evaluate where you stand.

Most people who live in the United States experience their hottest temperatures between mid-July and mid-August, meaning this holiday falls right in the thick of what is known as the *dog days of summer*.

While Americans have changed the meaning of the *dog days of summer* to refer to laziness in extreme heat, this was not the original meaning.

The *dog days of summer* originally referred to the astronomical event when the Greeks and Romans could see the bright star Sirius (from the Canis Major constellation) rising alongside the sun. They believed the closeness of Sirius to the sun was what caused the temperature to increase during this time. Canis Major (Big or Greater Dog) and Canis Minor (Lesser Dog) are the two constellations that follow Orion the Hunter across the night sky. The two dogs are his hunting companions. Hunting dogs, especially those belonging to a Greek giant would have been anything but lazy.

When you know the true origin of the phrase *dog days of summer*, you can see how the energies the Greeks and Romans associated with this time of year fit better with the true energies in nature than the laziness assigned to these days in more modern times. Lughnasadh is not a time of inaction. It is instead a time of a great deal of action with both harvesting manifestations and reevaluating goals and processes. Ancient civilizations could have been wiped out if they had not used the dog days for increased action instead of laziness and inaction. Work done on the hottest days of the year helped to keep people alive on the coldest. This blast of heat serves as a reminder the days are growing shorter; the time for action is now. The growing season is ending. It won't be long before the darkness of night overtakes the daylight. Winter is coming.

We can tap into the transformational energies of the dog days of summer while we evaluate goals and boost our manifestations.

For this ritual you will need:

- Representations of earth (salt, eggshells, or dirt), fire (candle), water (use your moon water), and air (incense or a feather)

- Lighter

- Spell or chime size candles in brown, gold, and orange with holders for each (placed in sand if necessary for safety)

- Ground cannabis (indica) to mix with the following in a blend:

    - Dried crushed skullcap

    - Dried crushed wormwood

    - Dried crushed thyme

    (This blend may also be made as a tea or in tinctures; prepare what you need ahead of time. If you are making a tea, you will need to have a pot of hot water and cup. If there isn't room for these on your altar, it is okay to leave them off, but place them close by.)

- Mortar and pestle

- Small spoon
- Small decorative container for your blend (You will make the blend as a part of the ritual.)
- Your ritual smoking piece, or supplies for your preferred method of consuming cannabis
- Comfortable way to sit on the ground, such as a meditation cushion or pillow
- Your journal, especially if you have a special one used for goals and manifestation tracking. Review any goal information you have documented before performing this rite.
- Something to write with

Optional:
- Any deity statues you would like to include and seasonal altar decorations

Set up your altar. You may use your own opening or the one included here.

Light your incense representing air and wave it around, allowing the smoke to whirl and swirl around you, or waft your feather and say:

> I call upon the spirit of air,
> Guide my intuition to see what lies before me.

Light the candle representing fire and say:

I call upon the spirit of fire,
Guide my mind to objectively see what lies before me.

Pour the moon water in a circle around your altar and sacred space and say:

I call upon the spirit of water,
Guide my heart to be open to what lies before me.

If you are using salt or dirt for earth and can sprinkle it on the ground around your altar and sacred space, do so. Say:

I call upon the spirit of earth,
Guide my will to be strong for what lies before me.

Take a moment to center and direct your focus. Invite your deity or deities to join with you or call upon your higher self by saying:

I call upon [name or archetype],
Guide me on the path, which lies before me.

Direct your attention to the three colored candles on your altar. As you light each one of the candles, take time to meditate on the qualities each of the colors is associated with and how these energies and qualities assist you on your journey.

Brown brings with it stability and balance. It helps us with concentration and focus, along with courage and decision-making. Gold energies encompass awareness and abundance. Intuition and illumination. Power and prosperity. Wisdom and well-being. Orange is an optimistic color flowing with creativity, encouragement, and transformation. All are key ingredients to objectively evaluate your work and make difficult decisions.

Knowing if a goal needs to be set aside or if you need to change your approach to succeed is as important as accomplishing the goals you complete. There are plenty of lessons where there is little to no success. Success, then, turns to learning these lessons for future wisdom.

Pause for a moment to refocus your mind on your next task: combining and mixing your blend together in the mortar and pestle. After you grind each herb, empty the mortar into your chosen container. Once they are all ground, you can either blend them together in the mortar or the container, whichever allows you the room to do so. If you are using tinctures, add as many drops of each as you want to your container to blend. Add cannabis, skullcap, and wormwood to the mortar and begin grinding and blending. (Keep the thyme on your altar but do not add to the blend yet if you are preparing your blend for smoking. When smoking thyme, a little goes a long way. If you are making a tea or tincture, it is okay to add it now.) As you work, say:

> *Guide me on this journey,*
> *With this blend I make.*
> *Guide me on this journey,*
> *I now prepare to take.*

Add your cannabis blend to your sacred piece, or prepare your preferred method of consuming cannabis. If you're smoking, top off with just a pinch of thyme to gently cover your blend. Thyme not only gives this blend a wonderful rich flavor, but it also brings with it many of its own special energies to help you achieve your task.

Seat yourself in a comfortable position to consume your blend (with as many refills as necessary, each time topping with thyme) and perform the following meditation. (If you are concerned you may drift off to sleep, use some modern magic and set a timer to wake you in about twenty minutes.)

> *Slow your breathing. Inhale for a count of five, hold for a count of five, exhale for a count of five. Take a moment to relax, ground, and center. Feel the energies of the herbs in your system.*
>
> *Allow the mundane world to fall completely away. Let any walls that surround you dissolve.*

Connect with your higher self. Feel yourself at one with the universe. Call to your deity if you desire.

Shift to the point of view of your higher self. Do this by becoming the narrator of your own story. Look at yourself from outside yourself, from your higher viewpoint. Describe how you see yourself sitting below, deep in meditation. Keep yourself in this perspective throughout this working.

Recall the list of objectives you have been working on for the year. Mentally check off any goals you have already achieved. Gather your harvest. Acknowledge the work and effort put into completing those tasks. Give yourself admiration and appreciation for the fruits of your labor. Wrap yourself in a hug if you wish. Praising yourself can be difficult, particularly if you aren't used to receiving it. Remind yourself you deserve it.

Are any of your goals unattainable or outdated? It happens. Don't feel bad. Simply remove them from your list. Goals can be revamped or modernized whenever necessary. They are not written in stone nor pledged with blood. They are guidelines and can be changed any time it becomes necessary. Priorities and outlooks change; goals can too. What once may have been an excellent idea may not be

anymore. File them away in your mind for reevalua-
tion later or toss into your mental trash bin.

Move down your list, reviewing your progress
with each goal. Is the goal attainable with its cur-
rent path? If not, could a new approach be helpful,
and if so, what? Think outside of the box. This is
a time when your creativity can flow in ways you
may not be used to. Like a hunter, you may need to
adjust your strategy to capture the prey. Ideas that
spring into your mind may surprise you with their
ingenuity. The energies and spirits you have called
upon are here to help you concoct new ideas, strat-
egize solutions, and dig for deeper revelations. They
will let you know when they have finished conveying
their message to you.

Open your eyes and write everything you can remember in your journal while it is still fresh in your memory. The longer you wait, the more information you may lose. Stand and stretch whenever needed.

To dismiss, recenter your focus one last time. Release your deity or deities by saying:

I thank you, [name or archetype],
For your guidance on my path.

Release each of the elements, saying:

I thank the spirit of air,
For your guidance on my path.

I thank the spirit of fire,
For your guidance on my path.

I thank the spirit of water,
For your guidance on my path.

I thank the spirit of earth,
For your guidance on my path.

My will be done.

While Lughnasadh is a harvest festival, it also represents rebirth and renewed ideas. There is still work to do and time to do it, but take heed—the darkness is coming.

MABON/AUTUMNAL EQUINOX

The autumnal equinox (known in some traditions as Mabon) is the true beginning of fall. It is the second harvest festival and a time when, once again, daylight and darkness are relatively equal.

From now until spring, the dark stretches further into the light, shortening each day until we reach the longest night of the year at Yule in a few months. More of our harvest has ripened. More of our goals are completed. It's time once again to inventory what we have achieved and give thanks for all that we have. This is when we celebrate the bounty of our harvest and work on tying up loose ends on projects that are almost completed. What still needs to be accomplished? What may have to wait until a later time? What achievements do you need to celebrate or give thanks for? What manifestations have you harvested?

A gardener uses this time to check plants to see what can be saved and encouraged to grow more before the end of the season. New flowers or fruits developing now will drain the plant of energy, which can be directed into salvageable fruit instead by pinching off the buds or fruits that will not ripen before the growing season ends. Do any of your goals need to be sacrificed for another to succeed? Cull anything you need to remove from your list for now. Focus your energies on the tasks that need your attention and successful cultivation the most.

The energies at the autumnal equinox are comparable to those at Lughnasadh, particularly with both being harvest festivals. The equinox gives us the extra reminder of the importance of balance in our lives. Work and play must be in equal measure. We did a bit of harvesting and cleanup work at Lughnasadh, which means after a brief spiritual check-in with the universe on where we stand with goals, it's time to celebrate the bounty and abundance of the year with the giving of thanks. The energies around us are shifting once again. We have had plenty of time to work on goals and for our gardens to grow. While there is still a harvest to gather, the time of rest is in sight. It is time to prepare for the cold days ahead when the energies turn from outer to inner workings. Mabon is often described as Pagan Thanksgiving, and with good reason. It's time to be thankful and reap the rewards of our hard work.

For this ritual you will need:

- Representations of earth (salt, eggshells, or dirt), fire (candle), water (moon water), and air (incense or a feather)
- Lighter
- Ground cannabis to mix with the following in a blend:
    - Dried crushed white sage
    - Dried crushed motherwort
    - Dried crushed holy basil (tulsi)

        (This blend may also be made as a tea or in tinctures; prepare what you need ahead of time. If you are making a tea, you will need to have a pot of hot water and cup. If there isn't room for these on your altar, it is okay to leave them off, but place them close by.)

- Mortar and pestle
- Small spoon
- Small decorative container for your blend (You will make the blend as a part of the ritual.)
- Your ritual smoking piece, or supplies for your preferred method of consuming cannabis
- Comfortable way to sit on the ground, such as a meditation cushion or pillow

Optional:
- Any deity statues you would like to include and seasonal decorations

Set up your altar. You may use your own opening or the one included here.

Light your incense representing air and wave it around, allowing the smoke to whirl and swirl around you, or waft your feather and say:

> *I call upon the air*
> *To join with me in this rite of thankfulness.*

Light the candle representing fire and say:

> *I call upon the fire*
> *To join with me in this rite of thankfulness.*

Pour the moon water in a circle around your altar and sacred space and say:

> I call upon the water
> To join with me in this rite of thankfulness.

If you are using salt or dirt for earth and can sprinkle it on the ground around your altar and sacred space, do so. Say:

> I call upon the earth
> To join with me in this rite of thankfulness.

Take a moment to center and direct your focus. Invite your deity or deities to join with you or call upon your higher self by saying:

> I call upon [name or archetype]
> To join with me in this rite of thankfulness.

Pause for a moment to refocus your mind on your next task: combining and mixing your blend together in the mortar and pestle. After you grind each herb, empty the mortar into your chosen container. Once they are all ground, you can either blend them together in the mortar or the container, whichever allows you the room to do so. If you are using tinctures, add as many drops of each as you'd like to your container to blend.

As you add each herb to the mortar, focus on the energies you want to call forth from it. The white sage cleanses, and it also helps you connect to your higher self while in a meditative state. Motherwort supports openness and self-love. Holy basil is associated with balance (perfect for an equinox), and it helps to restore energy—a bit of an extra boost. Add as much cannabis as you like into the mortar and begin grinding and blending. As you work, say:

Guide me on this journey,
With this blend I make.
Guide me on this journey,
I now prepare to take.

Add your cannabis blend to your sacred piece, or prepare your preferred method of consuming cannabis. Seat yourself in a comfortable position to consume your blend (with as many refills as necessary) and perform the following meditation. Set a timer if you wish.

Slow your breathing. Inhale for a count of five, hold for a count of five, exhale for a count of five. Take a moment to relax, ground, and center. Feel the energies of the herbs in your system.

Allow the mundane world to fall completely away. Let any walls that surround you drop away. Connect with your higher self. Feel yourself at one with the universe. Call to your deity if you desire.

Shift to the point of view of your higher self. Become the narrator of your story. Look at yourself from your higher viewpoint.

Recall the list of objectives you have been working on for the year. Mentally check off any more goals you have completed since Lughnasadh.

Move down your list, reviewing your progress with any goals you have left to complete—a quick check-in to see where you are. A cursory glance over your garden. You know what, if anything, you have left to finish. There's still time. Nothing to worry about today.

Recenter yourself, then turn your attention to the concept of thankfulness.

Look back over the past year and acknowledge any moments when you should have been more thankful than you were. Send the energy out now for what you missed before. Recognize what you take for granted. Note to be more appreciative when merited in the future.

Conjure up memories of gratitude, especially ones from the past year. Big or small. Every moment of thankfulness you can recall, grab onto the energy from each memory and infuse it into a bubble around you. Fill your bubble with these energies of appreciation until it feels as if the bubble will burst.

Float on these energies like bobbing on a raft in the ocean. Relax in your gratitude. Ride the waves of thankfulness.

It feels good to be thankful and grateful, yet too often, we take things, people, situations, even places, for granted. The saying "You don't know what you've got until it's gone" is often too true.

Make a vow to be more attentive to acknowledging your own thankfulness, not only now during the season for it but all year round. When you can, pay it forward with generosity from the heart.

When it is time to leave your bubble, center and redirect your focus. Release your deity or deities by saying:

I thank you, [name or archetype].
Your presence has been appreciated.

Release each of the elements, saying:

I thank the air for your energy.
Your presence has been appreciated.

I thank the fire for your energy.
Your presence has been appreciated.

I thank the water for your energy.
Your presence has been appreciated.

I thank the earth for your energy.
Your presence has been appreciated.

If you look through books or charts of correspondences, some of the qualities you will often find missing include ones such as thankfulness, generosity, and appreciation. While there are flowers that represent some of these types of energies, we don't have a whole lot that symbolizes these qualities. It is an area that feels as if it has been ignored or forgotten. It is important to make sure we create and put these energies to use, keeping them alive. The more thankfulness and generosity each one of us puts into the universe, the less apathy and greed there will be.

SAMHAIN

Most people celebrate this day as Halloween, the day when children dress up in costumes and go door-to-door asking for candy and other treats. It's a time for fun and a bit of mayhem, as ancient traditions have taken on modern-day twists. Haunted houses are major attractions as people pay for the privilege to be scared out of their wits by ghosts, demons, and other creatures of the dark. Spirits and monsters were once held at bay by the light of a carved turnip. Today people compete on TV shows for the best carved pumpkin.

Samhain, "summer's end," is filled with a wildly intense assortment of energies. It is the third and final harvest of the year. The fields are emptied, the growing season done. In olden times when a trip to the feed store wasn't a possibility, those who raised livestock had to decide how many and which animals to take with them through the cold months. Those not chosen for survival were slaughtered and salted for meat for the winter. Their sacrifice to help ensure the survival of the fittest animals is also known as a blood harvest. Though culling herds and flocks is still a reality in some agricultural families, it isn't something most people experience anymore.

Also known as the Witches' New Year, Samhain is the liminal time between the beginning of fall and the beginning of winter. The natural world around us has a completely different aura than what we felt at the equinox. It is no longer filled with life and activity. The leaves have all changed colors and fallen from the trees. Grasses have faded to yellow and brown. Birds have flown south for the winter, and small wildlife animals are curling up in dens and burrows for a long winter's nap. The nightly orchestra of crickets and frogs has ceased.

When plant life goes dormant, it no longer projects the same strong life force it does when healthy and in full bloom. With the sudden lack of life forces coming from the natural environment, humans become the strongest energy source, even when outside. This can be deceiving to those newer to the practice. While most witches may feel their powers increase at this time of the year, advanced practitioners also understand the decrease in natural energies in the environment may give false perceptions. The power that resides in you is more noticeable when there are not as many other energies available to camouflage it. Be sure you can tell the difference.

I believe spirits are more attracted to humans at this time of the year because human energy appears to be stronger with the lack of other natural competing life force energies. This also goes hand in hand with the thinning of the veil. The veil between our world and the Otherworld is thinnest at the time of year when the natural world is going dormant. Humans stand out like fireflies in a dark cave. Spirits are drawn to us like moths to a flame.

With all of this going on, it's easy to see how things might feel a bit off-kilter. You may find yourself a bit more "lightheaded" or even giddy. Your energy and abilities may feel overactive, or they may also feel fine-tuned. It's hard to predict ahead of time how the energy of this time of year will affect you, but chances are, you will feel different. You can sail through the Samhain season with blinders on and shut yourself down to noticing these changes, or you can open yourself to the opportunity of experiencing them and learning from them.

Samhain is the perfect time for learning how to distinguish and work with spirit energies. With the lack of present natural life force energies, spirit energy is easier for us to detect and register, just as it is easier for spirits to find our energy. In the summer months when life is full and vibrant, spirit energy is hidden, covered up. It comes across as a bit of static interference. But at Samhain, when the natural life force energies are dormant, the few still awake are the static interference while human and spirit energies reign supreme.

In this ritual, first you will evaluate and register your own power and energy levels. After that, your blend will help increase your energies to call in those who have departed. With the thinning of the veil, spirit communication becomes easier. What messages do your ancestors have for you?

A Samhain bonfire is the perfect accompaniment to a Samhain ritual, and if you are able to perform the ritual outside, the energies in the atmosphere will be even more easily felt and accessed. Remember, a small cauldron fire is a decent substitute for a bonfire.

For this ritual you will need:

- Representations of earth (salt, eggshells, or dirt), fire (candle, torch, or bonfire), water (moon water), and air (incense or a feather)

- Lighter

- Ground cannabis to mix with the following in a blend:
    - Dried crushed *Calea zacatechichi*
    - Dried crushed blue vervain
    - Dried crushed wormwood
    - Dried crushed mullein leaf
    - Dried crushed mugwort

        (This blend may also be made as a tea or in tinctures; prepare what you need ahead of time. If you are making a tea, you will need to have a pot of hot water and cup. If there isn't room for these on your altar, it is okay to leave them off, but place them close by.)

- Mortar and pestle
- Small spoon
- Small decorative container for your blend (You will make the blend as a part of the ritual.)
- Your ritual smoking piece, or supplies for your preferred method of consuming cannabis
- Comfortable way to sit on the ground, such as a meditation cushion or pillow
- Chime or spell size candles with holders: one black, one purple (along with a sand-filled platter for safety if desired)

- Journal
- Something to write with

Optional:
- Mary Jane magical mulch
- Cannabis kindling
- Cauldron or another fireproof container
- Any deity statues you would like to include
- Pictures of any ancestors or departed spirits you would like to connect with
- Seasonal decorations for your altar

Light your bonfire or cauldron fire, and set up your altar. You may use your own opening or the one included here.

Light your incense representing air and wave it around, allowing the smoke to whirl and swirl around you, or waft your feather and say:

> On this night when the veil is thinnest
> I call upon the spirit of air;
> Join with me in this rite
> And guide me on my path.

Light the candle representing fire and say:

On this night when the veil is thinnest
I call upon the spirit of fire;
Join with me in this rite
And guide me on my path.

Pour the moon water in a circle around your altar and sacred space and say:

On this night when the veil is thinnest
I call upon the spirit of water;
Join with me in this rite
And guide me on my path.

If you are using salt or dirt for earth and can sprinkle it on the ground around your altar and sacred space, do so. Say:

On this night when the veil is thinnest
I call upon the spirit of earth;
Join with me in this rite
And guide me on my path.

Take a moment to center and direct your focus. Invite your deity or deities to join with you or call upon your higher self by saying:

On this night when the veil is thinnest,
I call upon [name or archetype];

Join with me in this rite
And guide me on my path.

Pause for a moment to refocus your mind on your next task: combining and mixing your blend together in the mortar and pestle. After you grind each herb, empty the mortar into your chosen container. Once they are all ground, you can either blend them together in the mortar or the container, whichever allows you the room to do so. If you are using tinctures, add as many drops of each as you'd like to your container to blend.

Each one of the herbs you are using enhances spiritual connection and spirit communication. The astral realm is waiting for you.

Add as much cannabis as you like into the mortar and begin grinding and blending. As you work, say:

Guide me on this journey,
With this blend I make.
Guide me on this journey,
I now prepare to take.

Add your cannabis blend to your sacred piece, or prepare your preferred method of consuming cannabis. Seat yourself in a comfortable position to consume your blend (with as many refills as necessary) and perform the following meditation.

Slow your breathing. Inhale for a count of five, hold for a count of five, exhale for a count of five. Take a moment to relax, ground, and center. Feel the energies of the herbs in your system.

Allow the mundane world to fall completely away. Let any walls that surround you drop away. Connect with your higher self. Feel yourself at one with the universe. Call to your deity if you desire.

Shift to the point of view of your higher self. Become the narrator of your story. Look at yourself from your higher viewpoint.

On this night when the veil is thinnest, with natural energies dormant, it is easy to feel and recognize your own power. Light your black candle and take a moment to stare into the flame.

Burn away any impressions or conceptions in your mind. Let any thoughts burn up until all that is left for you to focus on is a pile of hot ash. As you stare at the pile, it begins to shudder and quake. A small light breaks through from below in a small fissure that appears. The heap of ash tremors more violently; more cracks appear, more beams of light.

You wait and watch for the eruption you know will occur.

The phoenix is reborn from the ashes. This one comes with a message for you, a true reflection of yourself. Listen to what the phoenix has to say. They know where your strengths lie, where your weaknesses lie. They know the power you hold and the power you do not. The phoenix will show you the expanse and the limitations of the power you possess. Listen well.

After the phoenix leaves, take time to breathe and recenter. Let the lesson sink in and fade away for now. Take another dose (or as many as you want) of your blend and refocus your mind on the next task at hand: lighting the purple candle and calling to the spirit realm.

Once it is lit, take some time to stare into the flame; let everything else fall away once again. Close your eyes and find yourself back in your bubble of comfort and safety.

Send out an invitation—who would you like to contact? DNA ancestors? Spiritual ancestors? A departed friend or family member?

If there is a specific spirit you would like to contact, call to them and invite them to join you. Understand "no" is an answer. You may not contact who you have called for. It is up to them if they want to come or not. Allow your guest(s) plenty of time to show. Trust in the process.

Whether your intended guest or another arrives, remind yourself this is their time. Let them communicate whatever message they have first. If there is time and energy left for questions, those can come after your visitor delivers their message. The "newer" a spirit is, the less experience they will have communicating with the living. Be patient. Trying to rush a spirit causes frustration, frustration causes interference, and interference means the communications aren't going to get through. This can go for emotions too; the more emotional you become, the more changes you are making to the energy field around you. This can be very disruptive to spirit communication. When you become more proficient at raising and sending energy, you can learn to funnel energy from yourself to the spirit to boost their signal.

When you are ready to end your spirit communication session, open your eyes and extinguish the black and purple candles. Take a moment to focus and recenter yourself.

Release your deity or deities by saying:

On this night when the veil is thinnest,
I thank you, [name or archetype];
Your presence in this rite
Guides me on my path.

Release each of the elements, saying:

On this night when the veil is thinnest,
I thank all the spirits who have joined with me.
I thank the spirit of air.
I thank the spirit of fire.
I thank the spirit of water.
I thank the spirit of earth.

Document in your journal who you spoke with and anything about the conversation you remember.

This ritual is best performed at sunset or midnight on October 31, but since the veil takes time to thin and then thicken again, you should get decent results for three days before and three days after, giving you ample opportunity to perform the ritual more than once if you wish.

Spirit communication takes an energy exchange with the Otherworld. It can be both exhausting and a bit addicting. Be sure to practice self-care and self-control.

YULE

The last of our sabbats is Yule, also known as the winter solstice and the longest night of the year. The natural world around us has gone to sleep. Plants are dormant and some animals have migrated while others have gone into hibernation. It is a time for rest and recovery.

Our energies turn from outer workings to inner workings. The first of those inner workings is the act of rest. Actual rest. Rest is not something common in a country where your value is so often judged on your measurable productivity. Sadly, if you are a woman, rest is often judged even more harshly.

Mother Nature herself takes a break from growing and being fertile and productive, but still, the concept of rest often gets a bad rap. Luckily, we know and understand that rest is an innate and intuitive action. It is a time to recover and store energy for use later during the growing season. The inner workings we do now prepare us for our outer workings, which come after the energy shifts again.

In this ritual, we will focus on resting and storing our energy. It is the longest night of the year, the perfect time to focus on rest. This ritual is best performed either at sunset on Yule or right before you go to bed.

For this ritual you will need:

- Representations of earth (salt, eggshells, or dirt), fire (candle, torch, or bonfire), water (moon water), and air (incense or a feather)
- Lighter
- Ground cannabis to mix with the following in a blend:
  - Dried crushed mugwort
  - Dried crushed peppermint

    (This blend may also be made as a tea or in tinctures; prepare what you need ahead of time. If you are making a tea, you will need to have a pot of hot water and cup. If there isn't room for these on your altar, it is okay to leave them off, but place them close by.)

- Mortar and pestle
- Small spoon
- Small decorative container for your blend (You will make the blend as a part of the ritual.)
- Your ritual smoking piece, or supplies for your preferred method of consuming cannabis
- Comfortable way to sit on the ground, such as a meditation cushion or pillow

Optional:

• Any deity statues or Yuletide decorations you would like to include

• If you like, a blanket to wrap up in

Set up your altar. You may use your own opening or the one included here.

Light your incense representing air and wave it around, allowing the smoke to whirl and swirl around you, or waft your feather and say:

I call upon the air in the east.
Lend me your power.
Lend me your sight.

Light the candle representing fire and say:

I call upon the fire in the south.
Lend me your power.
Lend me your might.

Pour the moon water in a circle around your altar and sacred space and say:

I call upon the water in the west.
Lend me your power.
Lend me your sight.

If you are using salt or dirt for earth and can sprinkle it on the ground around your altar and sacred space, do so. Say:

> I call upon the earth in the north.
> Lend me your power.
> Lend me your might.

Take a moment to center and direct your focus. Invite your deity or deities to join with you or call upon your higher self by saying:

> I call upon [name or archetype].
> Lend me your power.
> Join me tonight.

Pause for a moment to refocus your mind on your next task: combining and mixing your blend together in the mortar and pestle. After you grind each herb, empty the mortar into your chosen container. Once they are all ground, you can either blend them together in the mortar or the container, whichever allows you the room to do so. If you are using tinctures, add as many drops of each as you'd like to your container to blend.

Add a small spoonful of the mugwort into the mortar and say:

> Guide me to my sacred space.

Add a small spoonful of the peppermint and say:

Help me feel refreshed.

Add as much cannabis as you like into the mortar and begin grinding and blending. As you work, say:

Guide me on my journey,
With this blend I make.
Guide me on my journey,
I now prepare to take.

Add your cannabis blend to your sacred piece, or prepare your preferred method of consuming cannabis. Seat yourself in a comfortable position to consume your blend (with as many refills as necessary) and perform the following meditation.

Slow your breathing. Inhale for a count of five, hold for a count of five, exhale for a count of five. Take a moment to relax, ground, and center. Feel the energies of the herbs in your system.

Allow the mundane world to fall completely away. Let any walls that surround you drop away. Connect with your higher self. Feel yourself at one with the universe. Call to your deity if you desire.

Reflect on the natural world. Bring to mind the animals who have curled up to sleep off the win-

ter cold in their caves, dens, and burrows under the ground, or even in an old hollow tree. Think about the trees, now bare and dormant. Roots and seeds frozen in the ground, also frozen in time. They all know the importance of rest. The importance of taking the time for the self to rest and conserve energy.

How can you reflect this part of nature in your own life? How can you take the time to rest and conserve energy? What does this look like for you? Explore options and listen for messages from your deities or higher self. What recommendations do they have for you?

When you are ready to leave your sacred space, take a moment to center and redirect your focus. Release your deity or deities by saying:

I thank you, [name or archetype].
Your energy and power
Help me to succeed.

Release each of the elements, saying:

I thank the air of the east.
Thank you for your power.
Thank you for your sight.

I thank the fire of the south.
Thank you for your power.
Thank you for your might.

I thank the water of the west.
Thank you for your power.
Thank you for your sight.

I thank the earth of the north.
Thank you for your power.
Thank you for your might.

If you are not going to bed after this ritual, spend some time in a comfy spot, just staying warm and cuddled, like the bear in the den and the roots of the trees, resting deep under the frozen ground.

You are warm; you are safe.

It is time to let rest come.

Working with the Moon

While the sabbats deal with the energy changes throughout the year, we also experience energy from the moon, which fluctuates with its phases. (Think about the energy we experience daily; circadian rhythms have their own energy cycles too.)

While different pathways may vary slightly on how they interpret the phases of the moon, for the most part, they follow the same cycle. The new moon is a time of darkness, which means inner workings and rest, but also includes banishments of things we want out of our lives followed by new beginnings. As the moon waxes, we move toward a more active time of light, turning our attention to outer workings and bringing things into our lives.

The full moon has its own distinct energy. She is ripe and mature. Energy is at its peak of activity. As she begins to wane, we work on things we want to remove from our lives, aiming for them to be gone by the new moon. With this circular motion, we give ourselves time to complete short goals.

Waxing and waning, the moon gives us its own energy pattern for its lunar cycle. Adding cannabis to your moon workings gives you more energy at your disposal.

NEW MOON

While the focus and intent of each of your rituals will differ, this easy-to-follow blueprint helps you set and achieve your goals with the energy of a new moon.

For this ritual you will need:

- Bonfire or small fire in a fireproof cauldron or other container
- Representations of earth (salt, eggshells, or dirt), fire (candle, torch, or bonfire), water (use your moon water), and incense or a feather for air

- Lighter

- Ground cannabis (indica) to mix with the following in a blend:

  - Dried crushed rose petals

  - Dried crushed sacred lotus flower

  - Dried crushed hyssop

  - Dried crushed motherwort

  - Dried crushed mugwort

    (This blend may also be made as a tea or in tinctures; prepare what you need ahead of time. If you are making a tea, you will need to have a pot of hot water and cup. If there isn't room for these on your altar, it is okay to leave them off, but place them close by.)

- Mortar and pestle

- Small spoon

- Small decorative container for your blend (You will make the blend as a part of the ritual.)

- Your ritual smoking piece, or supplies for your preferred method of consuming cannabis

- Comfortable way to sit on the ground, such as a meditation cushion or pillow

- Chime or spell size candles in black and dark blue with holders

- Paper and writing utensil
- A journal to write your goals in

Optional:
- Mary Jane magical mulch
- Cannabis kindling
- Any deity statues you would like to include
- Your choice of music soundtrack and a way to play it

Set up your altar and light your fire. You may use your own opening or the one included here.

Light your incense representing air and wave it around, allowing the smoke to whirl and swirl around you, or waft your feather through the air and say:

> *I call upon the energy of air,*
> *Come to me this night,*
> *Join me in this rite.*

Light the candle representing fire and say:

> *I call upon the energy of fire,*
> *Come to me this night,*
> *Join me in this rite.*

Pour the moon water in a circle around your altar and sacred space and say:

I call upon the energy of water,
Come to me this night,
Join me in this rite.

If you are using salt or dirt for earth and can sprinkle it on the ground around your altar and sacred space, do so. Say:

I call upon the energy of earth,
Come to me this night,
Join me in this rite.

Take a moment to center and direct your focus. Invite your deity or deities to join with you or call upon your higher self by saying:

I call upon [name or archetype],
Come to me this night,
Join me in this rite.

Pause for a moment to refocus your mind on your next task: combining and mixing your blend together in the mortar and pestle. After you grind each herb, empty the mortar into your chosen container. Once they are all ground, you can either blend them together in the mortar or the container, whichever allows you the room to do so. If you are using tinctures, add as many drops of each as you'd like to your container to blend.

Rose helps us nourish our souls, gives us inner strength, and helps us with new beginnings. Sacred lotus intensifies our magic with its own. Hyssop helps us to remove stagnant or negative energies. Motherwort helps us to open ourselves to self-love and helps us to release emotional burdens. Mugwort, as always, helps us enter the spiritual realm.

Add as much cannabis as you like into the mortar and begin grinding and blending. As you work, say:

> Guide me on this journey,
> With this blend I make.
> Guide me on this journey,
> I now prepare to take.

Add your cannabis blend to your sacred piece, or prepare your preferred method of consuming cannabis. Seat yourself in a comfortable position to consume your blend (with as many refills as necessary) and begin the following meditation.

> Slow your breathing. Inhale for a count of five, hold for a count of five, exhale for a count of five. Take a moment to relax, ground, and center. Feel the energies of the herbs in your system.
>
> Allow the mundane world to fall completely away. Let any walls that surround you drop away. Connect

with your higher self. Feel yourself at one with the
universe. Call to your deity if you desire.

Light your black candle. We will begin by saying good-bye to anything we need to be rid of.

For your first new moon ritual, if you have not previously been working with lunar energies, you may not have anything you are ready to say a final goodbye to or goals that have been completed, so for your first ritual you may not have anything to do here. This may happen at other times too; it's okay if you have nothing to write down for a month. Simply skip over this part.

However, if you have already been working with lunar energies, then you may have a need for this part. You may also use a more cumulative approach for your first time and write down examples of recent goals accomplished or things you have recently successfully removed from your life. Use your paper and writing utensils to make the list of the things you are ready to say goodbye to.

When the list is complete, say:

This new moon signals the end of one phase
And the beginning of the next.
Tonight, the present becomes the past,
And then the future.
These things I now put behind me.

Light the paper on fire with the black candle and drop it into your bonfire, cauldron, or other firesafe container. As the list burns, each item moves into your past. Take a moment to "remove" the items on your list from your mind. Be sure to refresh yourself with more of your blend as needed.

Use the black candle to light the dark blue candle and then extinguish the black.

We move from endings and getting rid of the things we don't want in our lives to a bit of resting in the present. If you did not need to remove anything at this time, you will begin again here.

Close your eyes and redirect your focus to a mindfulness moment. Empty your mind of any other thoughts except for rest. Spend as much time here as you like, simply resting and being mindful of your music and the present. Feel yourself floating in your sacred space. Enjoy it for as long as you like. (Set an alarm beforehand if you are concerned about falling asleep.)

The new moon will soon begin waxing, growing stronger, brighter, and fuller each day. Use some deep breathing as you shift your focus from the present to working toward your future.

In your journal, write down whatever goals you have for the next two weeks. What new beginnings do you have in store for yourself? Phrase your goals in a way that shows they are progressing in a *waxing* manner. This may end up taking a bit of creativity. For example, imagine if your goals included something like weight loss or paying off debt. Normally these are things you would associate with waning, so you need to phrase these in a way that is waxing instead. "I add two pounds to my total weight loss." "I add one hundred dollars more to what I have paid off." Remember, these same goals can exist the other two weeks of the month during the waning period of the moon; they will simply be phrased differently when we continue to work with them after the full moon occurs.

Focus and phrase your intentions clearly. Finish the list and say:

> *This new moon signals the beginning of a new phase.*
> *As the moon waxes and grows,*
> *I look forward to the future.*
> *My intentions are set.*
> *My goals and plans*
> *Wax and grow*
> *Along with the phases of the moon.*

Set your journal aside, take another dose of your blend, and meditate on the achievement of your goals. Visualize your goals getting closer and closer to completion as the moon becomes fuller and fuller. Visualize what it looks like to have them fulfilled when the moon is full. Focus your intention and energy toward this vision becoming reality.

Spend as much time as you feel necessary in meditation and remember to set a timer if you are concerned about dozing off. Extinguish your candle when it is appropriate—either for safety reasons or to signify the end of your working.

Redirect your focus. Release your deity or deities by saying:

> *Thank you for your presence, [name or archetype],*
> *In my past, present, and future.*

Release each of the elements, saying:

> *I thank the energy of air*
> *For your presence*
> *In my past, present, and future.*
>
> *I thank the energy of fire*
> *For your presence*
> *In my past, present, and future.*
>
> *I thank the energy of water*
> *For your presence*
> *In my past, present, and future.*

I thank the energy of earth
For your presence
In my past, present, and future.

Magic doesn't "just happen." It is a focus of energy toward a specific intention. It gives your work in the mundane world a boost when the two are fashioned toward the same outcome. In turn, your work in the mundane world enforces your magical endeavors.

As we draw closer to the full moon, pay extra attention to see if you can feel the energy as it shifts.

FULL MOON

Our full moon rituals will follow a similar but rearranged pattern as what we did with the new moon, with the addition of time to raise and release energy with music and dance.

For this ritual you will need

- A space in which you may dance around safely
- Bonfire or small fire in a fireproof cauldron or other container
- Representations of earth (salt, eggshells, or dirt), fire (candle, torch, or bonfire), water (use your moon water), and incense or a feather for air

- Lighter
- Ground cannabis (you may want a hybrid, combination, or to alternate between indica and sativa; go with what works best for your purposes for each ritual) to mix with the following in a blend:

  - Dried crushed damiana leaf

  - Dried crushed California poppy

  - Dried crushed blue lotus flowers

  - Dried crushed mugwort

    (This blend may also be made as a tea or in tinctures; prepare what you need ahead of time. If you are making a tea, you will need to have a pot of hot water and cup. If there isn't room for these on your altar, it is okay to leave them off, but place them close by.)

- Mortar and pestle
- Small spoon
- Small decorative container for your blend (You will make the blend as a part of the ritual.)
- Your ritual smoking piece, or supplies for your preferred method of consuming cannabis
- Comfortable way to sit on the ground, such as a meditation cushion or pillow
- Your choice of music soundtrack and a way to play it

- Chime or spell size candles in dark blue and white with holders
- Your goal journal and a writing utensil

Optional:
- Mary Jane magical mulch
- Cannabis kindling
- Any deity statues you would like to include
- Drum, tambourine, or other handheld percussion instruments (you can use more than one throughout your dance)

Set up your altar and light your fire. You may use your own opening or the one included here.

Light your incense representing air and wave it around, allowing the smoke to whirl and swirl around you, or waft your feather through the air and say:

> *I call upon the energy of air,*
> *Come to me this night,*
> *Join me in this rite.*

Light the candle representing fire and say:

> *I call upon the energy of fire,*
> *Come to me this night,*
> *Join me in this rite.*

Pour the moon water in a circle around your altar and sacred space and say:

I call upon the energy of water,
Come to me this night,
Join me in this rite.

If you are using salt or dirt for earth and can sprinkle it on the ground around your altar and sacred space, do so. Say:

I call upon the energy of earth,
Come to me this night,
Join me in this rite.

Take a moment to center and direct your focus. Invite your deity or deities to join with you or call upon your higher self by saying:

I call upon [name or archetype],
Come to me this night,
Join me in this rite.

Pause for a moment to refocus your mind on your next task: combining and mixing your blend together in the mortar and pestle. After you grind each herb, empty the mortar into your chosen container. Once they are all ground, you can either blend them together in the mortar or the container, whichever allows you the room to do so.

If you are using tinctures, add as many drops of each as you'd like to your container to blend.

Damiana is uplifting and perfect for when we want to dance under and connect with the energies of the moon. California poppy adds its own dose of euphoria while blue lotus flowers also lift our mood. Mugwort helps us enter the spiritual realm. (This is one of my favorite blends!)

Add as much cannabis as you like into the mortar and begin grinding and blending. As you work, say:

> *Guide me on this journey,*
> *With this blend I make.*
> *Guide me on this journey,*
> *I now prepare to take.*

Add your cannabis blend to your sacred piece, or prepare your preferred method of consuming cannabis. Seat yourself in a comfortable position to consume your blend (with as many refills as necessary) and begin the following meditation.

> *Slow your breathing. Inhale for a count of five, hold for a count of five, exhale for a count of five. Take a moment to relax, ground, and center. Feel the energies of the herbs in your system.*
>
> *Allow the mundane world to fall completely away. Let any walls that surround you drop away. Connect*

with your higher self. Feel yourself at one with the universe. Call to your deity if you desire.

We begin by raising energy in the best ways there are: song and dance. Have a playlist ready to go. A slower song at the beginning before increasing the tempo helps to warm the body up. Build and release energy as much as you like, just don't wear yourself out too much, as we have more work yet to do.

There is something truly amazing about dancing in the dark under the full moon, particularly when you are incredibly high. It's a point of view not many people take the time to experience. Trust me, take the time as often as you can.

For this part of the ritual, I recommend either a hybrid or alternating between indica and sativa. After the dance, I would switch to straight indica to finish the ritual.

When you are ready to continue, light your dark blue candle and be sure it is in a safe location as we move on to a bit of resting in the present. Close your eyes and redirect your focus to a mindfulness moment. Empty your mind of any other thoughts except for rest. Spend as much time here as you like, simply resting and being mindful of your music and the present. Feel yourself floating in your sacred space. Enjoy it for as long as you like. (Set an alarm if you are concerned about falling asleep.)

To finish our working, use the dark blue candle to light your white candle and extinguish the blue. We end with harvesting what we have been working on since the new moon and set our goals to work on as the moon completes her cycle.

Review your goals from your journal. Were you able to check them all off? Any goals not yet completed should be written in a manner that coincides with the waning energies of the moon over the next two weeks, if you are going to continue with them. In our new moon ritual, we used the example of weight loss and paying off debts. Those same types of goals would now be written in a style of "I eliminate one hundred dollars of my debt." "I lose two pounds." Focus and phrase your intentions clearly. As the moon grows darker, your energy turns more inward and back toward rest. Be sure your goals reflect this.

Finish the list and say:

> *The full moon signals the beginning of a new phase.*
> *As the moon wanes,*
> *I look forward to the future.*
> *My intentions are set.*
> *My goals and plans*
> *Work with the phases of the moon.*

Set your journal aside, take another dose of your blend, and meditate on the achievement of your goals. Visualize your goals getting closer and closer to completion as the moon decreases. Visualize what it looks like to have them fulfilled when the moon is dark. Focus your intention and energy toward this vision becoming reality.

Extinguish your candle when appropriate to signify the end of your working.

Redirect your focus. Release your deity or deities by saying:

Thank you for your presence, [name or archetype],
In my past, present, and future.

Release each of the elements, saying:

I thank the energy of air
For your presence
In my past, present, and future.

I thank the energy of fire
For your presence
In my past, present, and future.

I thank the energy of water
For your presence
In my past, present, and future.

I thank the energy of earth
For your presence
In my past, present, and future.

———

Working with the energy cycle of the year and the lunar phases is an incredibly powerful way to live your life in balance with nature. We often hear about living our lives in balance with work and being sure to leave some time for fun, but this isn't what balance really is at all. The only balance that truly matters is when we live our lives in balance with nature. When we work with nature instead of against it, we discover our own true meaning of life. The answers are all right there waiting to be found.

Working with weed and the energies of the year helps us to recognize and feel energy shifts, even when subtle. Better perception of energy leads to better control, focus, and direction. These abilities open the doors to many worlds, opportunities, and adventures. Once proficiency is achieved in these skills, you will also have achieved a different outlook on life.

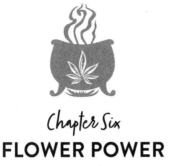

Chapter Six
FLOWER POWER

There is no denying the power of the flower is strong in many ways. It is healing, it is uplifting, it can transport us to alternate worlds and connect us to our gods. Weed weds us to the natural world. This bond gives our abilities and power immense potential. You can change your world and the world around you. You simply must want to and work at it. It won't change to what you want without your help.

In this chapter, we will go over a few more ways to add an extra boost to your conjuring and then move on to more specific spells and rituals for a better, more in-touch-with-nature-and-yourself life.

Get into Your Groove

Witchcraft is serious business, but there is plenty of room for joy, celebration, and, on occasion, a bit of absurdity. Laughter and high jinks create and emanate positive energy. Brightening your practice with cheer and merrymaking instills its own positivity into your workings. Performing serious work in an ecstatic, enthusiastic, and elevated manner gets the job done and produces its own positive energies. In some cases, like attracts like: when we send out positive energies to others and to the universe, we attract more positivity into our own life.

When you have fun and enjoy your practice, you are more likely to actually participate in a practice. I have heard hundreds of times why some witches do not follow through with their practice:

- "I know I should meditate, but I just don't have the time."
- "I should do a ritual for the full moon, but I have nothing prepared."
- "I can't keep track of when the new moon is."
- "What is the full moon good for again? The new moon?"

You may have used some of these excuses yourself; I know I have. The thing is, when your practice is fun, you make the time. When your practice is fun, you look forward to working with the energies of the new and full moon so you are better prepared and you commit.

We are conditioned to believe that serious matters require a certain solemness to them, and while this is true for some occasions, it does not have to be for all. With the witch population explosion that accompanied the COVID-19 pandemic, many of them came from a variety of Christian backgrounds where the solemness during religious or spiritual events was emphasized. It's simply true: witches do have more fun.

As witches, we work with the natural energies in our universe, and we know joy, happiness, and laughter are incredibly powerful natural energies, so let's have some fun.

Dance Like No One Is Watching

Like many little girls, I was enrolled in dance at a very young age with my mother's hope I would someday become a famous ballerina. I clearly remember my first pink leotard with pink tights, pink ballet shoes, and black tap shoes that were so much fun to walk in and make a racket with. Problem was, I was far more interested in the sounds I could make than dancing. Ballet didn't stick. I tried "jazz" dance the summer after seventh grade, but one thing was made perfectly clear to me: I couldn't dance. Not well anyway. I wasn't Elaine from *Seinfeld* bad, but there was no way a career as a dancer would be in my future.

Fast forward to present day, and now I find myself running women's dances under the full moon in The Spiral Labyrinth.

I still can't dance very well and will even trip over my own feet frequently. The difference now is why I am dancing. I'm not dancing to learn new steps. I'm not dancing to appease the wishes or expectations projected onto me by someone else. I'm not dancing to impress a romantic interest. I'm not dancing for anyone but myself. I am dancing for the endorphin boost. I am dancing to feel a connection to the trees, birds, grass, and flowers. I am dancing to feel a connection to the full moon ripe in the night sky. I am dancing to feel a connection with the other women who join me. I am dancing to feel a connection with the goddess and with the universe.

You do not need to be a great dancer to enjoy the power of dance. All you really need is to do it. Dancing can be elaborate or simple—tapping your feet to the beat and waving your arms while still seated both count in my book. Physical limitations need not exclude you. Don't focus on what you can't do; focus on what you can.

Combining dance with weed will bring different results depending on the weed and the music you are using. Ensure your weed matches your mood, desire, and intention.

Faster, upbeat music for energy raising goes well with sativa strains. Indica strains are more in touch with soft, ethereal music. You can focus on one ambiance or alternate between them. Begin with an energy-raising sativa and dance, and then finish off with a slow, grounding, leisurely indica and whirl. Experiment with different songs, different strains, and different types of dances. Rituals and spellwork can be easily edited to include music and dance to help raise, focus, and release energy.

Dance helps you to feel better about yourself, and feeling better about yourself makes you feel more like dancing. It's a win-win.

Music is a universal power. It conveys emotions and messages. It guides us to build energy, release it, and ground ourselves afterward. Whether we are dancing, singing, or both, music is spiritual.

Sing Like No One Is Listening

I sing even worse than I dance, but it doesn't stop me. In fact, it encouraged me to include song in my practice once I realized it doesn't matter if I can't carry a tune. The use of my voice raises energy. The use of my words raises energy. The speed at which I sing can increase or decrease energy. I have incredible control over energy with my voice. So do you. Of course, having a talent or developed skill for singing is wonderful, but don't feel you have to be worthy of an audition on *The Voice* to use your voice to sing or chant in your practice.

We often have no problem singing along to the radio in our cars, but when we go to sing in a spiritual manner, we freeze up. It may be a new experience for you, which can be a bit intimidating. Simple chants are great for beginners. Listen to witchy- and Pagan-themed music and learn the words just as you do with the songs on the radio. One of the greatest advancements I have seen in the Pagan world in the past three decades is the amount of and easy access to Pagan music. Not using it would be a shame. Spells, rituals, meditations, divination sessions, and any other crafting purposes can all be made more powerful with music. Using your voice in song in your practice is an effective energy amplifier.

Remember how weed has this great way of lowering walls you have built up around you? This helps us to relax and release anxieties we may have about singing in a spiritual manner.

It's important to add here, for some people, singing in a spiritual manner is a trigger. This is particularly true for "newer" witches who have also been deconstructing trauma sustained through their religious upbringing. I have had conversations with several people who have experienced this, as I had myself. Once you understand this trigger and work through it, you can take back your voice to build new memories in which you relish singing into your power.

Flying in the Forest

"Forest bathing" is a Japanese concept that has gained popularity the world over, though many cultures understand the importance of the nature-human connection. Sadly, not all cultures do. American culture has pushed that exhaustion from work or play is an ideal state of mind. It isn't. You don't have to work harder and play harder to be happy. You do have to learn to take care of yourself and give yourself what you need to be happy.

Spending time in nature is essential for good mental health. Essential. We need it. When we cut ourselves off from nature, we suffer from it. Give yourself and your mental health what you need by taking the time to get yourself out into a place of nature. Whether it is a huge forest, small country park, or a tree in your own backyard, make the time to get out there to sit or lie down and "bathe" with the trees.

Pick out a scenic, quiet location and get yourself comfortable. You may use a chair, pillow, blankets—whatever you need to make yourself cozy. Be sure to have some music ready and headphones if you need them. Remember, if you are in a place where smoking isn't ideal, there are other methods of consumption (edibles, RSO, tinctures) available. Also, if you are afraid you might doze off, don't forget to set an alarm.

Before you consume any cannabis, tune in to the natural world around you using as many of your senses as you can. Feel the ground and grass beneath you. Smell the air. Taste the breeze. Listen to the wind, the leaves rustling; what other sounds do you hear? Lie down and look upward into the leaves. Absorb everything around you. Tune in to the world around you as much as you can, then consume your cannabis; give it time to take effect, and then again, reach out to the world around you, focusing on one individual sense at a time. Feel the ground below you again. Smell the air, taste the breeze, listen to the wind. Feel the connection deepen. Relax, breathe, and simply enjoy the use of your senses and all your experience.

Try forest bathing at different times—a morning experience will be far different than one in the afternoon or one late at night. Your senses will be able to pick out many differences, and you will encounter various energies.

Getting high in nature is one of my favorite activities. I have a large swing (one I can lie down on) next to the labyrinth, which I get high on and commune with nature. It is peaceful, restful, and restorative—all qualities we need to be at our best. For me, a peak experience while forest bathing pretty much sums up the best parts of life.

Stream of Consciousness Writing

Made popular by authors such as James Joyce and Virginia Woolf, stream of consciousness writing had its start in psychology. Used to describe the inner monologue some people have, it is a way to get everything that is floating around in your head down on paper, and sometimes the results may be surprising.

The prompts here are ones to help increase and boost positivity in your life. I recommend using a hybrid, combining indica and sativa strains, or alternating back and forth between them while working with stream of consciousness writing. You may answer a question with different strains and find it gives you very different answers. These questions are designed to get you started free-flow writing. You can also do this by recording yourself talking and then listen back to it or by typing on a device, but pen to paper adds its own sort of energy. Electronic devices can be distracting, especially if notifications go off. Experiment to find out what works best for you.

Get as high as you comfortably can and still be able to perform the tasks you need to, such as writing or typing. You do not want to zone out mid-sentence (which is why sativa may be helpful) of what could be an important statement.

Stream of consciousness writing can be done freeform (without a prompt) or with one of the prompts listed below.

When you are done writing, read it over to see what stands out to you, making any notations you want to add (use a different colored pen), then set it aside and read again later when you want.

Writing Prompts

- My favorite aspect of myself is…
- My earliest favorite memory is…
- I am happy when…
- When I am happy, I…
- What I liked about my childhood (teen years) was…
- The first time I remember being proud was…
- Positive things I tell myself are…
- I feel generous when…
- I feel safe when…
- My best trait is…

Focusing on the good aspects of your life gives them more energy. These writing prompts can help you create a bit of positivity anytime you need it.

SIMPLE BREATHWORK MEDITATION

Meditation is a long-standing practice with untold benefits for the body, mind, and spirit. Modern researchers have studied this ancient practice to discover how it reduces stress and anxiety and promotes both emotional and even physical health. When thinking about what a meditation practice may look like, many conjure images of clear minds, peaceful humming, harmonic chanting, and tuning out the outside world for hours at a time to find enlightenment. Although this may be reality for some dedicated practitioners, a modern meditation practice can look much simpler yet still provide the same physical, emotional, and mental health benefits.

Meditation is not just about releasing the busy thoughts rolling around in your mind; it is also about breathing deeply and allowing your lungs to fully expand as you inhale oxygen and fully release as you exhale carbon dioxide. Breathwork is an important part of meditation and is a big reason why meditation is so beneficial for the body. This breathwork can help strengthen lung power and improve overall lung capacity.

The goal of this simple breathwork meditation is to take a few minutes out of your day to turn your attention inward and release any tension that you may be holding onto because of stress and anxiety while also strengthening your lungs with your breath. This works best with smoking, dabbing, or vaping. Release any negativity and replenish yourself with positivity. Deep breathing, especially when accompanied by a big bowl of weed or a fat doobie, can instantly take you from a mundane realm of negativity to a spiritual world of positivity.

This meditation can be practiced in any safe location. All that is important is that you are comfortable and have a few moments to yourself.

When you are ready to begin, smoke, vape, or dab your weed and close your eyes. Breathe normally for a moment and pay attention to how it feels as you inhale and exhale. Take note of any place where you feel movement and where you feel any tension. Now take the breath deeper. Slowly inhale through your nose, allowing the belly to expand, fully filling your lungs with air. As you exhale, the belly should slowly release. The focus here is to transition from shallow "chest breathing" to a deeper, fuller breath using the diaphragm. With true "belly breathing," the diaphragm pushes your organs down, causing the belly to expand, then draws the organs back upward to push carbon dioxide from the body. This is the good stuff—this is where many of the physical benefits of meditation come from, and this is the part of the practice that helps to improve lung capacity.

Take a few moments here to notice how the full diaphragmatic breath feels in your body. When you feel ready, begin to count the inhalations and the exhalations. Start by inhaling for four counts and exhaling for four counts. After a few rounds, expand the exhalation to six counts. This may take some practice, but when you feel ready for the full cycle, focus on expanding your exhalation to eight counts. The goal is to inhale deeply through your nose for four counts and exhale fully for eight counts. Spend as much time here as you need.

As you become proficient at this breathing practice, add in smoking with some of the inhalations. Experiment with spacing out how often you smoke. When done for an extended period of time, this process can get you extremely high. Have your lemon oil and coffee beans close by to sniff in case you need them. Being this high may also lead to nausea or vomiting. Be aware of side effects you may experience. This breathing process has lifted me into a peak experience many, many times, and I willingly confess it has also involved tossing my cookies on most of those.

You may find yourself becoming distracted by the thoughts that pop up. This is okay! Simply take note of the thought and release it to return to the breath. Distractions, whether external or internal, are a normal part of life and a normal part of any meditation practice. The goal is to return your focus back to the meditation and the present moment. Meditation is not sitting still with a completely blank mind, but training your mind to refocus your attention and awareness.

If you go high enough into a peak experience, your higher self will take your thoughts where they need to go.

You can spend as little or as long as you like on this meditative practice and can return to it as often as needed. This can be part of a daily routine practice or just an exercise that you turn to in a time of need. Remember, this is your practice and your journey, so do what is best for you and your lifestyle.

SELF-LOVE BATH SPELL

Self-love is an important step on any spiritual journey. It can also be very difficult to give yourself love, especially if you are a female who was programmed to believe women are supposed to take care of others, even to their own detriment. This is a belief that women have worked decades to overcome. Sadly, we are seeing a resurgence of it in our own political system. Everyone deserves self-love. Everyone.

Prepare your bathwater before you begin the ritual. If you choose, you can set the mood with some relaxation music or your favorite empowering songs.

For this spell you will need:

- Small slip of paper
- Writing utensil
- Tea light candle

- Ground cannabis (indica) to mix with the following in a blend:

    – Dried crushed sacred lotus flower

    – Dried crushed rose petals

    – Dried crushed motherwort

    (This blend may also be made as a tea or in tinctures; prepare what you need ahead of time. If you are making a tea, you will need to have a pot of hot water and cup.)

- Lighter or match

- Mortar and pestle

- Small spoon

- ¼ cup of a skin-nourishing base—for the base you can use colloidal oatmeal or your favorite bath salt such as Epsom salts, pink Himalayan salt, or sea salt

- Small dish to prepare your bathing mix

- ½ tablespoon chamomile

- ½ tablespoon pink rosebuds or petals

- Your ritual smoking piece, or supplies for your preferred method of consuming cannabis

- Strainer to catch the herbs and petals

Before you begin, you will need to prepare the tea light candle with your intention. First, take the slip of paper and your writing utensil and write a short petition. This can be something personal related to your intention, or you can use your favorite self-love affirmation. This petition can be as simple as "I love myself." Choose whatever feels best for you. Write down your intention and then fold the slip of paper toward yourself three times to draw your intention to you.

Next, you will take the tea light candle out of its aluminum holder and place the petition in the holder. Sprinkle a tiny pinch of your herbs and petals on top of the petition, then cover it up with the tea light candle.

Once your candle is ready, light it. You can call to any deities or your higher self if you choose as you prepare your blend and bathing mix.

Place a spoonful each of sacred lotus flower, rose petals, and motherwort into your mortar. If you are using tinctures, add as many drops of each as you'd like to your container to blend.

Each of these herbs helps us to give loving care to ourselves. Add as much cannabis as you like into the mortar and begin grinding and blending. As you work, say:

> Guide me on this journey,
> With this blend I make.
> Guide me on this journey,
> I now prepare to take.

Set this blend aside to work on your bath blend.

Pour the quarter cup of oatmeal or salt into a small dish and add your chamomile and rosebuds on top. Close your eyes and focus on your intention as you stir the mixture clockwise.

When you are ready, draw the bathwater to your desired temperature, then pour the mixture into the bathtub and mix it around with your hands. Enter the tub, find a comfortable seat, and, cupping your hands, scoop up water to pour over your body.

When ready, place your blend in your piece or use your preferred method of consuming your blend, and relax. Let yourself get into a comfortable state of mind.

Recite your intentions out loud; this sends your words out to the universe while also affirming these intentions to yourself. You may recite whatever you wrote down on your petition for the candle. Truly speak from the heart and don't hold anything back.

After you have finished and you feel that you have no more to say, end your petition with these words:

> *I am worthy of and deserving of self-love.*
> *I love myself for who I am,*
> *Today and now,*
> *Forever and always.*

Dose again if you like. Relax and enjoy the time you have alone. This ritual can be repeated as often as you like or made a part of your weekly routine.

When you are finished with your bath, use a strainer to collect the herbs and petals you have used to avoid clogging the drain. Return the herbs and flowers to the earth. Allow the candle to burn out fully on its own if you can, even if you do not remain in the bath that long.

SELF-LOVE ROSE QUARTZ SPELL

Rose quartz has long been related to self-love practices due to its associations with compassion, inner peace, and nurturing positive emotions. With this spell, you will be charging a rose quartz with your intentions for self-love and positivity.

You can use any rose quartz crystal of your choosing, whether it is rough or tumbled, small or large—it is entirely up to you. A palm stone or rose quartz jewelry are excellent options as well. After completing this spell, the rose quartz can be worn, carried with you, or placed on your altar.

You can also use this spell to charge rose quartz that will be used for other purposes, such as with the Self-Love Spell Jar coming up next. All the herbs used in this spell are also used for the Self-Love Spell Jar, so the two workings can be combined into one ritual if you choose.

For this working you will need:

- Small dish or bowl

- Pink Himalayan salt

- Charcoal tablet

- Lighter

- Cauldron or other firesafe container

- Ground cannabis (indica) to mix with the following in a blend:

    – Dried crushed rose petals

    – Dried crushed lavender buds

    – Dried crushed thyme (just a pinch)

    – Dried crushed holy basil (tulsi)

    – Dried crushed lemon balm

    (This blend may also be made as a tea or in tinctures; prepare what you need ahead of time. If you are making a tea, you will need to have a pot of hot water and cup. If there isn't room for these on your altar, it is okay to leave them off, but place them close by.)

- Mortar and pestle

- Your ritual smoking piece, or supplies for your preferred method of consuming cannabis

- Pink rose petals or rosebuds

- Lavender buds

- Thyme

- Basil

- Lemon balm

- Any kind of rose quartz

Before you begin this spell, set your intentions and call upon your guides. Fill the small dish or bowl with your pink Himalayan salt so that it is ready for you at the end of the spell. Light your charcoal tablet within your cauldron or other firesafe container so that it sparks and is ready for the dried herbs.

Mix your blend together with the mortar and pestle. I recommend heavier on the rose petals and lavender and lighter on the other herbs, but this is a matter of taste only. Once prepared, smoke yourself into your comfortable sacred space. (Or use your tea or tinctures.)

Focus and speak your intentions out loud. Say:

Love for self,
And love divine,
I am worthy and deserving,
Of what is mine.

Take a pink rose petal or rosebud and drop it onto the charcoal tablet to burn and say:

Rose so pink,
Help me blossom to my best self.

Add a sprinkle of the lavender buds to the charcoal tablet and say:

Buds of lavender, provide peace and harmony,
Aid me in my journey.

Next, add the thyme to the cauldron and say:

As thyme burns, my courage and strength grow.

Drop the basil onto the charcoal as you say:

Basil, banish negative self-talk,
As I promote compassion, loyalty,
And harmony within myself.

Finally, add the lemon balm to complete the incense as you say:

Lemon balm, lift me up;
I attract success in my spell and love for self.

Allow the incense to burn and take the rose quartz into your hands. Carefully hold it over the cauldron, allowing the smoke of the incense to charge the crystal with your intentions. Close your eyes and imagine a warm and loving light emanating from the crystal as you repeat the opening incantation once more:

> *Love for self,*
> *And love divine,*
> *I am worthy and deserving,*
> *Of what is mine.*

When you have finished, leave the crystal in the dish of pink Himalayan salt to continue charging and let the incense burn out on its own. If you have extra herbs left over, you can use them for the Self-Love Spell Jar or sprinkle them into the bowl of pink salt.

SELF-LOVE SPELL JAR

Spell jars have recently become an increasingly popular form of witchcraft. They are versatile, simple to create, and easily customizable—not to mention, they certainly fit a witchy aesthetic. I love spell jars for long-term or even permanent spellwork, so a spell jar for self-love is an excellent way to utilize this trendy form of spellwork.

For this spell, you will need a glass jar. Any kind of jar will do if it has a lid that can be sealed tight. Something with a screw top or cork would do nicely. Your jar can be as large or small as you like as long as it will fit all of your ingredients. I often use crafting jars, and there are many budget-friendly options available at dollar stores as well.

Once your jar is filled with your ingredients, you will want to seal it with wax. There are two ways of doing this: you can burn a pink candle, allowing the wax to drip down, or you can use a wax melt commonly found in wax seal kits. Scented wax from a wax lamp is also an option if you have the means to pour the wax over the top of the jar safely without burning yourself. If you are not interested in using any form of hot wax, you can wrap the top of the jar with pink ribbon.

This spell uses the same ingredients and intentions as the self-love rose quartz spell, and the two can be combined into one ritual if you choose. The self-love rose quartz spell can be used to charge the ingredients that you will use here, and the same incantations will be used to simplify this process.

For this working you will need:

- Ground cannabis (indica) to mix with the following in a blend:
    - Dried crushed rose petals
    - Dried crushed lavender buds
    - Dried crushed thyme (just a pinch)

- Dried crushed holy basil (tulsi)

- Dried crushed lemon balm

     (This blend may also be made as a tea or in tinctures; prepare what you need ahead of time. If you are making a tea, you will need to have a pot of hot water and cup. If there isn't room for these on your altar, it is okay to leave them off, but place them close by.)

- Mortar and pestle

- Your ritual smoking piece, or supplies for your preferred method of consuming cannabis

- Lighter

- Pink Himalayan salt

- Any type of glass jar with a lid

- Small piece of paper

- Writing utensil

- Rose quartz

- Pink rose petals or rosebuds

- Lavender buds

- Thyme

- Basil

- Lemon balm

- Pink candle or wax melt

- Optional: pink ribbon

Before you begin this spell, set your intentions and call upon your guides. You may cleanse the jar ahead of time if you choose.

Mix your blend together with the mortar and pestle. I recommend heavier on the rose petals and lavender and lighter on the other herbs, but this is a matter of taste only. Once prepared, smoke yourself into your comfortable sacred space. If you are using a tea or tincture, take it now.

Begin with the pink Himalayan salt to cleanse and charge your ingredients. After adding the salt to the jar, take your paper and writing utensil and write out your petition and intentions. You can include any runes or personal sigils and symbolism that you use as well. When ready, fold the paper three times toward you to attract your intention to you. Hold the paper with your petition in one hand and take the rose quartz in your other and recite these words out loud:

Love for self,
And love divine,
I am worthy and deserving,
Of what is mine.

Tuck the paper into the jar and add the rose quartz as well. Take a pink rose petal or rosebud and add it to the jar as you say:

Rose so pink,
Help me blossom to my best self.

Add a sprinkle of the lavender buds to the jar and say:

Buds of lavender, provide peace and harmony,
Aid me in my journey.

Next, add the thyme and say:

As I add thyme, my courage and strength grow.

Add the basil to the spell jar:

Basil, banish negative self-talk,
As I promote compassion, loyalty,
And harmony within myself.

Finally, add the lemon balm as you say:

Lemon balm, lift me up;
I attract success in my spell and love for self.

After you have added your last ingredient, it is time to close and seal the jar, using either the pink candle or wax melt or the pink ribbon. Once the jar has been sealed, use this final incantation to seal your intentions to the spell:

I love myself for who I am.
I am worthy of love.

I am deserving of love.
I am love divine.

Your spell jar can be carried in your purse, placed on your altar, or kept in another safe place.

Cannabis is an amazing and versatile ingredient in the recipe for a happy life. Not only can it help us find joy and peace and bring a smile to our faces, in the tough times, through the hard work, cannabis lends a hand to help guide us through. We will learn how in our next chapter on shadow work.

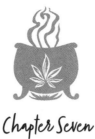

Chapter Seven
SHADOW WORK

I wrote an article for the *Llewellyn's 2023 Witches' Companion* about cannabis and shadow work, so I am pleased to be able to expand on the topic here.

To begin, we must first do some groundwork and discuss safety concerns. Let's begin with what shadow work is and what it isn't.

Shadow work is a form of psychoanalysis in which the practitioner looks at the repressed, hidden aspects of their self to heal and learn from past traumas and experiences to integrate all parts of the self into one. It is a tool used in psychotherapy practices all over the world. It can be done with or without a therapist, though a therapist is highly encouraged. Only you know if you are ready to work through the aspects of your shadow self. No one else can judge that for you. Never allow anyone to push or guilt you into shadow work you are not ready to perform. If at any time you find yourself in a distressing situation, seek professional assistance immediately.

Shadow work can be extremely triggering, which is why it is often done with a therapist. It may bring about repressed memories which, when remembered, can feel as if the trauma is happening for the first time. Therefore, it is important to work at your own pace and do so in a safe manner when and how you are ready. Only you know when you are capable of facing the hauntings and traumas of your own past.

The end goal—integrating all your parts together to make a whole complete person—is an ongoing, never-ending process. We learn. We get better. We do better. And sometimes we screw up again, and we start over to figure out why. We keep going. We learn. We get better. We do better.

Witches know that when one can work with and control all aspects of their self, they are better able to control outside forces, including the manipulation of energies. This makes our power, well, more powerful.

Shadow work is not something only used by witches, no matter what WitchTok says. Shadow work is useful for everyone and anyone who wants to use it. Witches may be drawn to it more than others due to their very nature as healers. Healers want to be whole and healed. They may also be drawn to it more because of the power it gives them as they heal. Finally, because it has been talked about in the witch community through social media so much in recent years, some people have classified shadow work as a necessity to be a witch. This is simply not true. There are plenty of witches with no interest in shadow work. Their pathway is their pathway, as yours is yours. No one can dictate your path, and you cannot dictate the path of anyone else. This is true for everyone. We each have a unique journey to follow. Our paths are our own.

Let's turn now to discussing how and why cannabis is so helpful with shadow work.

Unlock Your Mind

Weed is a key to unlocking your mind, which makes it highly beneficial in shadow work. When used at an optimum dosage, cannabis allows the user to step aside and see themselves from their higher self's viewpoint. This is a component of a peak experience: the blissful state a person reaches when they feel at one with the universe and can see themselves and their actions from an objective point of view. During a peak experience, cannabis gently lowers the walls of defense the psyche has built up around you and cradles you in comfort as revelations are unveiled. A peak experience is a safe space, but you must know how to access it to use it to its full potential. You must also be capable of coping with the aftereffects of learning what you discover. For more in-depth information on peak experiences than what we previously covered here, I urge you to please read *Wake, Bake, and Meditate* before delving too deep into the world of shadow work if you are still new to cannabis. The best preparation work beforehand will give you the best results within your shadow work practice. Learn how to fully use the tools and skills at your disposal.

When walls come down, repressed memories may be one of the shadows that come through. I have recovered memories through peak experience shadow work. Several of these memories were traumatic and painful in themselves. With these memories, certain implications may occur regarding the divulged memory. The "how" and "why" these traumas occurred, along with how they were handled in real time by others close to us, can be as daunting as the original trauma, creating more matters of contention. Therefore, it is important to understand both what you can deal with on your own and where your limits abide. It is also important to keep in mind, false memories are also possible.

Increased anxiety with cannabis use can be a real problem. The uncovering of suppressed memories can trigger anxiety, particularly after exiting a peak experience. It is important to know how you react in these kinds of situations before you are in one and how your cannabis use may affect anxiety. Emotional coping skills are essential. Being able to pull yourself out of the experience (with the aid of smelling coffee beans or an essential oil, or using a large dose of CBD) is also essential. If you are unsure if you can do this on your own, don't. Practice with a trusted partner present first.

You may remember some ordeals too well, with the memory itself being what led to the shadowed trait. You may understand precisely where a shadowed trait came from but need more work to help you identify how to heal from the trauma. Shadow work allows us to revisit traumatic events with an arsenal of tools we were not equipped with the first time around. Damage remains until we heal it. Often when trauma occurs, we don't have the skills at the time to cope with it, especially if it happens during childhood. It takes maturity, growth, and understanding to learn the skills needed to cope and heal. Shadow work provides the opportunity to use learned information and skills to heal past traumas.

Not all shadow work should be done in a peak experience, but it is extremely helpful for certain exercises. Anytime you use cannabis, it helps to lower your defensive walls and see yourself and your actions from an objective viewpoint. We will begin with gentler exercises before moving on to those of a more in-depth nature where a peak experience is desirable.

Get in the Zone

Shadow work requires preparation. You don't just decide, "Oh, I have ten minutes to spare, time for a little shadow work." It requires commitment, willingness, and advanced preparation.

Let's begin with where you do your shadow work. Your location needs to be a place where you feel safe and comfortable. You may have several places you work, but they will all need to be places where you are completely at ease. You may prefer to do your shadow work in a dimly lit room where shadows are easily visible. Or you may desire a spot near a window where the sun shines brightly on your face in symbolism of bringing your shadow self to the light. Contemplate what environment works best for your healing. What do you need?

Add to your atmosphere to boost your experience: incense, oil diffusers, pillows, candles, blankets, fresh flowers, plants. Make the spaces you use places of healing. When you can, work outside in nature.

You will also want a journal specifically for your shadow work. Pick something nice to use, like one of the many gorgeous journals you have stashed on a shelf but then don't use because they are too nice. Shadow work is the perfect time to use a "special" journal because healing is incredibly special. Spoil yourself for the work you are going to undertake. You deserve it.

Obviously, you will also need cannabis in whatever form you prefer to take it. Be sure to have enough available for extra doses.

Thanks to TikTok, the question has been raised of whether you should use protective magic during shadow work. Shadow work is a therapeutic tool and does not require divine protection nor intervention. Shadow work deals with the hidden aspects of yourself. Aspects that have been hidden by an ego trying to protect you. Asking for protection during shadow work would then be counterproductive. Think about what it is you are wanting protection from—yourself? What dangers do you believe exist in looking inside yourself? Feeling a need for protection may be a sign you are not yet ready to explore certain aspects of your shadow self and should try exploring areas that do not feel as threatening.

Taking Inventory

We will begin with a gentle journal exercise. You will want to be comfortably high but still capable of writing—don't go 110 percent couch potato. Allow yourself to feel lifted, comforted, safe. Take a few moments to breathe deeply and slowly. Relax.

Mindfully bring yourself into the moment. A trick to doing this is to imagine yourself "stepping back" and seeing what you are doing and thinking. Become your own witness. This helps separate your thinking self from your higher self. An example of how to do this: my thinking self is lying on my couch typing these words right now onto my laptop. But I can stop for a moment, "step back," and let my higher self see I am thinking and working. For me, when I make this switch, I go from thinking *I* to thinking *she*. This may help you make the transition.

Once you step outside of yourself, you can see yourself from an objective viewpoint. The walls are gone. You can see yourself more clearly than ever before. You can see your positive traits and you can see the negative ones. Spend as much time as you need adjusting to seeing yourself from this new point of view. If you have not taken a good objective look at yourself before, this process can be startling and even a bit shocking when you discover things you didn't know were there.

When you are ready, begin writing out two lists. The first list is your positive traits and qualities, the second list your negative ones. Alternate between the two as you take an inventory of how your higher self sees you. You aren't being hard on yourself. There is no guilt, no shame—only objectivity. You are finding where your flaws lie to help heal the traumas that created them.

Take extra doses as you work to easily stay in your higher self. When you feel you are done, set your journal aside. Take several deep breaths and relax. Let yourself enjoy and ride out the rest of your high. If you are feeling sad or low, recall a favorite memory to focus on as you come back down. Reward yourself for your hard work.

A large part of shadow work is finding the shattered pieces, cleaning them up, and putting them back together again. These lists give a starting point for deeper shadow work while also reminding yourself what you have to be proud of.

Remembering the Past

Not all childhood traumas are hidden with repressed memories. There may be events that happened that are incredibly clear in your mind and play over repeatedly. These acts of trauma at a young age create trauma response behaviors that attach to your personality. Trauma responses are classified in four different categories: fight, flight, freeze, and fawn. While some trauma response behaviors come from repressed events, others are born with our full memories intact. We will work with what we remember first. Have your journal close by.

Choose a memory you feel ready to explore and dose yourself into a comfortable state.

Think back to the event you have chosen and remember the details, as much as you are comfortable with at this time. Remind yourself as you recall any distressing details, you are safe. You are no longer in the situation. You are only observing it. Nothing can hurt you. Nothing can harm you. Tell yourself this as often as you need it.

Walk yourself through the following questions, writing your answers in your journal:

- What damage did this trauma cause you?
- What was your response?
- What were the responses of others?
- How have you coped with this event since it happened?

Unfortunately, wishing an event never happened doesn't do anything to help us cope with it, learn from it, and move on. Trying to forget doesn't help if we haven't healed the trauma first. These are both forms of denial. The trauma responses remain until they are healed. What does help is learning to accept what happened, healing from it, and putting ourselves back together to live our best and healthiest life.

When trauma happens to us as children, we often do not possess the skills to help us cope with it. We may not even possess the communication skills to seek out help or explain the trauma we have suffered. We rely on those who care for us to respond in a way that makes us feel better, safe, and protected. However, we don't always get the response we want or need, and this may leave us unable to heal for quite some time. Sometimes those who are supposed to protect us are the ones who hurt us most.

What do you need to help yourself heal from the damage that was done?

Give yourself what you need. This can include realizing and accepting your own innocence. Through gaslighting and other methods, children can be conned into believing acts of violence or neglect committed against them were their own fault, which causes its own set of trauma responses.

Tell yourself what you wanted to hear. Give yourself the support you wanted to have but did not receive. Cry if you need to. Take your time and heal. Wrap yourself in a tight embrace and hold it for as long as you like. Write about your experience in your journal when you are ready.

Repeat this meditation for remembered traumas when you are ready to work through them. Don't feel discouraged if you feel the need to work through a traumatic event more than one time. It may take several sessions to work through some experiences others only take one. Everyone and every experience is different.

Stream of Consciousness Writing

Stream of consciousness writing has great potential for helping to uncover the shadow self, especially when you are in an elevated state of mind and spirit with your defenses lowered. When the walls come down, the truth comes through.

I recommend using a hybrid, combining indica and sativa strains, or alternating back and forth between them while working with stream of consciousness writing. You may answer a question with different strains and find it gives you very different answers. These questions are designed to get you started free-flow writing. You can also do this by recording yourself talking and then listen back to it or by typing on a device, but pen to paper adds its own sort of energy. Electronic devices can be distracting, especially if notifications go off. Experiment to find out what works best for you.

Get as high as you comfortably can and still be able to perform the tasks you need to, such as writing or typing. You do not want to zone out mid-sentence (which is why sativa may be helpful) of what could be an important statement.

Stream of consciousness writing can be done free-form (without a prompt) or with one of the prompts listed below. When you are done writing, read it over to see what stands out to you, making any notations you want to add (use a different colored pen), then set it aside and read again later when you aren't stoned. Keeping a journal of these writings can help you discover and work through a variety of problems along the journey of your shadow self.

Writing Prompts

- If I could change one thing about myself at the snap of my fingers, I would change…
- My earliest memory is…
- If I could change one thing about my past, I would change…
- I get sad when…
- When I get sad, I…
- I get angry when…
- When I get angry, I…
- I lied when…
- What I didn't like about my childhood (teen years) was…
- Something I want to forget but can't is…
- I have never talked about…
- I count on other people to…
- When I am disappointed, I…
- The first time I remember being disappointed was…
- I don't know how to meet my needs of…

- Negative things I tell myself are…
- I feel guilty about…
- I need to forgive myself for…
- I feel anxious when…
- I don't feel safe when…
- I get scared when…
- When I get scared, I…
- My worst trait is…
- I feel alone when…
- My parents' worst traits are/were…

Writing about these traumas and negative aspects brings your shadow self to the surface, where it can be exposed to light and healed. These writings give you road maps to follow in your healing journey.

BURN IT ALL DOWN CORD CUTTING SPELL

Cord cutting spells are a great tool for severing ties to other people, negative traits and behaviors, or unpleasant situations. When it comes to shadow work, cord cuttings are about releasing ties to anything that may be holding you back in your spiritual practice as well as in your life. Once these cords have been cut, you may find more freedom in your shadow work practice. This cord cutting spell focuses on severing energetic ties to fear, negative self-image, and anything else that you feel may be holding you back.

For this working you will need:

- Ground cannabis (sativa) to mix with the following in a blend:
    - Dried crushed motherwort
    - Dried crushed thyme

        (This blend may also be made as a tea or in tinctures; prepare what you need ahead of time. If you are making a tea, you will need to have a pot of hot water and cup. If there isn't room for these on your altar, it is okay to leave them off, but place them close by.)

- Mortar and pestle
- Your ritual smoking piece, or supplies for your preferred method of consuming cannabis
- Two pieces of paper and a writing utensil
- Two taper or chime candles, preferably white or one white and one black
- Firesafe plate or tray
- A flammable cord or string, about nine inches long
- White salt
- A lighter
- Journal and pen

Before you begin this ritual, it is important to make sure that you will not be disturbed and that you are in a safe space where you feel comfortable. Shadow work practices can leave you feeling vulnerable as you begin to work within yourself. Know that this practice is completely on your terms and that you can always pause your practice and return to it later. Working at your own pace is very important; take as much time as you need.

This ritual will be set up with two candles connected by string surrounded by a circle of white salt. One candle will represent you and the other candle will represent all that you are releasing and cutting ties to. If you are using two different colors, use the white candle for yourself and the black candle for what you will be releasing.

Prepare your blend by grinding and mixing the motherwort, thyme, and cannabis together. This combination helps us to receive our own self-care while also protecting us from what we are working to sever. We use sativa for this spell, as its energy is more like the energy of fire than indica's energy, and we are using fire to sever ties. Add the mixture to your ritual piece and smoke yourself into your desired state. If you are using a tea or tinctures, make your blends and take them.

When you are ready, take the two slips of paper, one for each candle, to solidify your intentions. On the first piece of paper, take a few moments to write out your strengths, shadow work goals, and the positive aspects of yourself that you embody. Place this piece of paper in front of or underneath the candle representing you. On the second piece of paper, write out all that you wish to cut ties with. This can include your fears, negative traits and behaviors that may be holding you back, intrusive thoughts, and negative thought processes that you feel may be slowing your progress. Place this piece of paper in front of or underneath the second candle, both on the firesafe tray.

Once the candles are prepared, take the cord or string and wrap it around the first candle three times. Leave some slack and wrap the other end around the second candle three times. The cord represents the energetic connection that will be burned away. Don't forget to use a firesafe plate or tray and create a circle of white salt around the candles and your petitions.

You may call upon any higher power or spirit guides to assist you in this working as you take a few moments to set your intention. Consume more of your blend anytime you feel it is necessary. Focus on each candle, close your eyes, and see in your mind what each candle represents to you. After your intentions are set, light the wick of each candle, starting with your candle. You can speak your intentions out loud, ask for the energetic connections to be severed as the cord burns away, or sit in quiet reflection.

As the candles burn down, the cord will eventually catch fire and burn away. Keep a close eye on the cord and flame to ensure your safety. Do not leave this ritual unattended for any reason, as it is a fire hazard. Allow the cord and both the candles to burn out completely on their own. After they do, finish your spell with the words:

What is gone never shall return.

SAVE IT FOR LATER SHADOW WORK SPELL JAR

Though we often see them being used for a type of banishing, spell jars can be used in a variety of ways. The key to a spell jar is that it contains or restrains something. Jars can be sealed so whatever is inside stays there, or the top may remain removeable. This allows you to take out what is in your jar later. This will be the basis for our spell jar.

Spell jars can be extremely useful in shadow work, particularly if you ever find yourself overwhelmed. Need a break from all that is on your mind? Write it down and stick it in a jar. Uncover several shadow side traits at once and don't know which one you should start working with first? Stick them all in a jar and pull one out when you are ready. Jars are a good, safe place to keep things we know we need to deal with but don't want in our minds on a constant basis. One of the keys to successful shadow work is timing. Timing and knowing yourself well enough to understand your own limitations and reactions is crucial. If you know that certain topics are extremely triggering for you, you may not be ready to work on them. Stick them in a jar until later. Pushing yourself when you don't feel ready is at least counterproductive and can be dangerous to your mental stability. If you don't feel ready, you aren't. When you are ready, you will know. The desire overcomes the fear.

For this spell you will need:

- Glass jar with an airtight lid large enough to fit your herbs, stones, and rolls of slips of paper (You can get a bit creative here—you will be keeping this jar, so if you want to make it special or unique somehow, do it!)

- Moon water

- A cleansing incense stick, such as frankincense or sage, and holder

- Lighter

- Ground cannabis (indica) to mix with the following in a blend:

    - Dried crushed white sage (just a pinch, as it's strong)

    - Dried crushed rose petals

– Dried crushed motherwort

(This blend may also be made as a tea or in tinctures; prepare what you need ahead of time. If you are making a tea, you will need to have a pot of hot water and cup. If there isn't room for these on your altar, it is okay to leave them off, but place them close by.)

• Mortar and pestle

• Small spoon

• Your ritual smoking piece, or supplies for your preferred method of consuming cannabis

• A pinch of any (or all) of the following herbs to help control and diffuse: chamomile, lavender, valerian, or vervain

• Any (or all) of the following stones to help control and diffuse: amethyst, bloodstone, carnelian, chrysocolla, fluorite, or howlite

• A pinch of any (or all) of the following herbs to help release anxiety: bergamot, frankincense, jasmine, lemon balm, pennyroyal, or wormwood

• Any (or all) of the following stones to help release anxiety: agate, chrysoprase, or hematite

• Small slip(s) of paper

• Writing utensil

To begin, be sure your jar is physically clean and rinse with your moon water. Allow it to air dry.

Light the incense stick and insert the lit end into the jar and swirl it around three times, cleansing the jar. Say each time:

> *I cleanse this jar,*
> *Negativity be gone.*

Set the incense in the holder and place out of your way.

Add the white sage, rose petals, and motherwort to your mortar with as much cannabis as you like and begin grinding and blending. As you work, say:

> *Guide me on this journey,*
> *With this blend I make.*
> *Guide me on this journey,*
> *I now prepare to take.*

Add the blend to your sacred piece and smoke yourself into a comfortable state. If you are using a tea or tinctures, make your blends and take them. To build your jar, begin with the herbs you selected from the first category—those to help control and diffuse. Take a pinch of each one you're using and add it to your jar. Say:

> *This herb I add has its own power.*
> *Keep what is inside over the hours.*

As you add the herbs, imagine the power of the herbs keeping the issues and their effects inside of the jar. While they sit there, the strength of the issues will diffuse. It will become less, making the issues easier to deal with.

Add each of the stones to help control and diffuse and say:

> *This stone I add has its own power.*
> *Keep what is inside over the hours.*

Again, imagine the power of the stones adding to the power of the herbs, diffusing the strength of your shadow traits.

Add the herbs you selected from the second category— those to help release anxiety. Take a pinch of each one you use and add it to your jar. Say:

> *This herb I add has its own power.*
> *To weaken my shadows over the hours.*

As you add these herbs, imagine them helping to release anxiety that these shadow traits cause within you.

Add each of the stones to help release anxiety:

> *This stone I add has its own power.*
> *To weaken my shadows over the hours.*

Imagine the power of the stones adding to the power of the herbs, releasing any anxiety these shadow traits hold over you.

Anytime you feel you need it, take more of your blend.

Using the strips of paper, write down keywords, phrases, and sentences related to the events and issues you know are there but you aren't ready to work on quite yet—anything you need to put on hold and temporarily out of your mind. Or, if you have several issues to deal with and don't know where to begin, write each one down on a separate slip. When you are done writing, roll each one into a tiny scroll and say:

> I roll you up
> To pack away
> And revisit again
> Another day.

Drop each scroll one by one into the jar. Say:

> Into the jar
> I place you now,
> To revisit again,
> This I vow.

After filling the jar, place the lid on tightly. Know that what is in the jar is still an unhealed part of you. Place it near a window where it will receive both sunlight and moonlight. The energies of the herbs and stones work to neutralize the issues you have stuck in the jar.

When you are ready, pull a scroll from your jar to begin working and healing through the problem.

CANNABIS COFFIN CREMATION BANISHING SPELL

Let's talk about the difference between banishing and binding. You may have your own ideas and definitions, so let me explain my view so you see where I stand, so you may better choose which most suits your needs.

To be blunt, *banishing* is permanent: finished, *finito*, done, over, outta your life, gone for good. A *binding* does not have to be permanent. Bindings can be removed. Bindings are used in situations where a banishing may be too extreme. This working is for things you want or need completely out of your life. This can include anything from negative habits to negative people. This spell packs the unwanted into a coffin with a small cannabis offering, which is all then cremated. Let's begin!

For this spell you will need:

- Bonfire or small fire in a fireproof cauldron or other container. (It needs to be large enough to contain the fire from burning the cauldron.)

- Lighter
- A small wood coffin (available at craft stores)
- Black paint or a thick black permanent marker
- Ground cannabis (indica) to mix with the following in a blend (and a pinch for an offering):
    - Dried crushed white sage (just a pinch, as it's strong)
    - Dried crushed mugwort

        (This blend may also be made as a tea or in tinctures; prepare what you need ahead of time. If you are making a tea, you will need to have a pot of hot water and cup. If there isn't room for these on your altar, it is okay to leave them off, but place them close by.)

- Your ritual smoking piece, or supplies for your preferred method of consuming cannabis
- Mortar and pestle
- Small spoon
- Small slip(s) of paper
- Writing utensil
- Frankincense or myrrh resins (or both)
- Florida water

Optional:

- Mary Jane magical mulch
- Cannabis kindling

Set up your altar and light your fire.

Prepare ahead of time:

- Paint or color the coffin black, both inside and outside.
- Prepare your smoking blend and have your piece ready to go.

Write down the things you want to banish from your life. Be very focused and precise with your wording and intent, and be very sure this is what you want. Save this type of working for the worst of the worst.

Roll up the strips of paper and place inside the coffin along with the frankincense, myrrh, or both and a pinch of cannabis as an offering. This offering is to help send what you have written down away in peace, no matter what it is. You want it gone, so let it go in peace. Close the clasp on the coffin.

Holding the coffin away from your body, carefully and slowly pour Florida water over it, both sides. Try not to get it on you, as it is highly flammable. While you pour, say:

> *What is inside this coffin*
> *Is gone from me and my life.*

Focus your attention on the flames in the fire and the way they consume everything in their path. The fire burns it all away, turning everything it touches to ash. Toss the coffin into the fire.

Light your blend and smoke (or drink your tea or tincture) while you watch the coffin burn. Meditate on what your new life looks like.

MALICE IN CHAINS BINDING SPELL

As stated previously, bindings can be temporary. A binding can be released if you so wish. They are a good way to help temporarily control a situation, trait, event—whatever it is you need control over. For our purposes, we are referring to aspects of your shadow self. There are many different ways you can use a binding spell. You can use it to bind issues you aren't ready to deal with. You can use it to bind personality traits you are working on controlling—even the urge for a cigarette, drink, or candy bar can be bound.

In this spell, we will use the power of intention to charm a chain for temporary bindings. The chain is for you to wear, as it will be binding these things inside of you.

For this spell you will need:

- Small fire in a fireproof cauldron or other container—you will be passing the chain through smoke, so you will want to keep the fire small

- Lighter

- Your ritual smoking piece, or supplies for your preferred method of consuming cannabis

- Ground cannabis (indica)

- Any of the following herbs ground together, prepared ahead of time to burn: black pepper, clove, cypress, dragon's blood resin, High John root, mandrake, pine, rosemary, willow, or wormwood

- A chain of your choosing

Optional:
- Mary Jane magical mulch
- Cannabis kindling

Set up your altar, light your fire, and smoke yourself to your comfortable space. If you are using a tea or tinctures, make your blends and take them. Keep your fire small and slowly add your herb mixture to it. Be mindful of how much you use at a time. Too little and you might not get enough smoke if your flames are too big. Too much and you may suffocate the fire if the flames are too small.

Once you have smoke, focus on your intention—precisely what you are binding—and pick up your chain.

Carefully, hold the chain in the smoke of the herbs. Be careful not to burn yourself. Visualize the power you and the herbs are instilling into each link of the chain, each one becoming stronger, each one entrusted with control. As you hold it in the smoke, chant:

> *This chain I enchant*
> *To bind what I must.*
> *When I wear it,*
> *The magic I trust.*

Continue chanting until the smoke is gone or you feel the chain is empowered. Wear it when you need it.

SHADOW WORK TAROT CARD SELF-REFLECTION RITUAL

For generations, tarot cards have been a favorite divination tool among witches and other spiritual practitioners. Not only for divination, tarot cards are also used to help gain insight and clarity as a therapeutic device, which makes them an excellent addition to your shadow work toolbox.

This ritual is intended to be repeated as part of your practice and may help guide you on your shadow work journey. Each time you perform this ritual, you will focus on a different card. How you decide the card you use is entirely up to you. You can work through the major arcana in order, shuffle the deck to be guided to a card at random, or look through and choose the card that calls to you. You have the choice of working just with the major arcana or using the full deck. If you don't work with tarot, this ritual can be performed using your favorite oracle card deck as well. Choose what is best for you; there are no wrong answers when it comes to this ritual.

Whichever deck you choose to work with, I recommend dedicating it to your shadow work practice until you are finished working through the cards. Remember to pull each card you complete from the deck so that you can progress through it.

For this working you will need:

- Your ritual smoking piece, or supplies for your preferred method of consuming cannabis
- Ground cannabis (indica) mixed with mugwort
- Lighter or matches
- A notebook or journal
- Pen or pencil
- A tall white candle
- A dedicated tarot or oracle card deck

Begin this ritual by smoking yourself into your sacred space. If you are using a tea or tinctures, make your blends and take them.

Call to your guides, deities, or other higher power to assist you and allow you to be open to the process. Have your writing utensil and journal or notebook ready, as this self-reflection ritual focuses on journaling.

When you are ready, light the white candle and set your intentions. For this ritual, you will speak your intentions out loud before you choose or reveal the card that you will be working with. While holding the cards in your hands, say:

> I summon my shadow self.
> I look within to gain insight and clarity.
> Cards of fortune, reveal to me where
> My work begins today.

Turn over the card that you will be working on today and take note of the immediate thoughts and feelings that come up. Write these down in your journal to reflect on. Allow yourself to free write. There are no wrong answers. Whatever comes up is a part of what you need to focus on in your journey. Allow yourself to connect to your shadow side instead of overthinking the topic with pre-written journaling prompts. With this practice, you are essentially creating your own writing prompts. Look over the card, connect to the images and what they make you feel. Is there something about the artwork that reminds you of something else? Journal about it and ask yourself why.

Next, you will connect with the meaning of the card—and yes, feel free to use the deck's guidebook for this one! What questions can you ask your shadow self that relate to the card's meaning? Are there any key words or phrases that call out to you? Write these down and reflect on what they mean to you.

Your shadow self will come through with messages for you to help you on your healing journey.

Shadow work isn't easy; it wouldn't be called *work* if it was. It isn't for everyone, but it is for those who are ready to face the negative aspects of life and work for a better future—both for themselves and the world they live in.

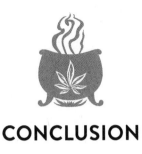

CONCLUSION

I have known since I was six years old that there was something different about me, a sign being when I knew my dog had died before my parents came to tell me. When they asked me how I already knew, I told them it was because she had come to say goodbye. Two years later, I had a similar experience when it was my mother's turn to say goodbye. It wasn't until I was sixteen that I learned about the concepts of channeling and mediumship.

Throughout the years and books, I have definitely had a bit of supernatural guidance with my writing. From helpful nudging tips to demanding screams of "Don't forget…!" there have been different assistants throughout my career. Cannabis has made the channeling process so much easier for me; it can sometimes be difficult to even realize when I am doing it.

My writing process has always been very similar to stream of consciousness writing. I write down whatever pops into my mind and hope it makes sense. When I am channeling, it can be difficult to type as fast as what I am hearing. Sometimes I have gone back to reread what I wrote and realized I had no recollection of putting those words down. In the past, however, the esoteric voices have focused on *writing*. This time, among my posse I found a new voice—one of an editor! I was repeatedly interrupted by this new voice telling me how to fix things, where to move things, or encouraging me to find a better word choice. (This particular paragraph has been a real doozy!)

Not only does cannabis offer greater power and focus for conjuring, but it also provides a conduit for more intense and productive channeling. Cannabis has long been used as a pathway to speak with spirits and deities. This power is easily obtained—when the cannabis plant is not regulated by governmental laws, that is. Perhaps this power, the power for people to take their spirituality and their divinity into their own hands, is another one of the reasons we are still in the battle over the legality of a plant.

We leave you with these last few words of advice: Your spirituality is *your* spirituality. Your path is *your* path. There is far more to the world than television shows, work, and social media. There is a world outside your doorway and an entire other world inside your mind. Cannabis can quite literally help you tap into both. Learning to work with it can change your entire outlook on life. I know it sure has mine.

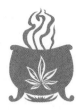

A NOTE FROM THE AUTHORS

Tyler has compiled several great playlists that can be used for many of the workings in this book. He has copied all those lists (and we will continue to update and add more) to a Spotify account under my name, Kerri Hope Connor. Enjoy!

To Write to the Author

If you wish to contact the authors or would like more information about this book, please write to the authors in care of Llewellyn Worldwide Ltd. and we will forward your request. The authors and publisher appreciate hearing from you and learning of your enjoyment of this book and how it has helped you. Llewellyn Worldwide Ltd. cannot guarantee that every letter written to the authors can be answered, but all will be forwarded. Please write to:

Kerri Connor
Tyler D. Martin
Krystle Hope
℅ Llewellyn Worldwide
2143 Wooddale Drive
Woodbury, MN 55125-2989

Please enclose a self-addressed stamped envelope for reply, or $1.00 to cover costs. If outside the U.S.A., enclose an international postal reply coupon.

Many of Llewellyn's authors have websites with additional information and resources. For more information, please visit our website at http://www.llewellyn.com.